Teaching Nutrition and Food Science

Teaching Nutrition and Food Science

Margaret Knight

B T Batsford Ltd London

© **Margaret Knight 1976**

First published 1976
ISBN 0 7134 3094 X (hard cover)
ISBN 0 7134 3099 O (limp cover)

Printed in Great Britain by
Biddles, Guildford, Surrey
for the publishers
B T Batsford Limited
4 Fitzhardinge Street
London W1H 0AH

Contents

Acknowledgment 8
Preface 9

1 INTRODUCTION TO NUTRITION AND FOOD SCIENCE 11

Basic chemical structure of foods
Chemical and physical changes occurring in food preparation   Osmosis
Diffusion   Solutions   Colloids   Emulsions   Suspensions
Acidity and alkalinity of food   *Practical work*

2 DIGESTION AND ABSORPTION 22

Digestion in the mouth   Digestion in the stomach
Digestion in the small intestine
Absorption of the nutrients in the small intestine
Absorption and utilisation of sugars   Absorption and utilisation of fats
Absorption and utilisation of proteins
Absorption of vitamins, minerals and water
Practical work on digestion
Summary of digestive enzymes

3 ENERGY 32

Uses of energy in the body   Calories and kilojoules
Basal Metabolic Rate   *Practical work*   States of energy imbalance

4 PROTEINS, FATS AND CARBOHYDRATES 43

The chemistry of proteins   The essential amino acids
The non-essential amino acids   Protein quality
Food sources of protein   Daily allowance of protein
Functions of proteins in the body   Signs of deficiency of protein
Practical work   Simulated meat protein
Fats   Phospholipids   Steroids   Triglycerides   Saturated fatty acids
Unsaturated fatty acids   Essential fatty acids   Daily allowance of fat
Functions of fat in the diet

Carbohydrates   Monosaccharides   Disaccharides   Polysaccharides
Average daily intake of carbohydrates
Functions of carbohydrates in the diet
Chemical tests for proteins, fats and carbohydrates

5   VITAMINS   58

Vitamin A   Hypervitaminosis A   Vitamin D   Vitamin E
Vitamin K   The B Complex   Vitamin B1 Thiamine
Vitamin B2 Riboflavin   Vitamin B3 Pantothenic acid   Nicotinic acid
Vitamin B6 Pyridoxine   Folic acid   Vitamin B12 Cyanocobalamin
Vitamin C Ascorbic acid   *Practical work*

6   MINERALS AND WATER   72

Calcium   Phosphorus   Sodium   Potassium   Magnesium   Iron
Trace elements   Iodine   Fluorine   Copper   Cobalt   Zinc
Practical work on minerals   Water   The role of water in nutrition

7   MILK   87

Composition of cow's milk   Identification of nutrients present in milk
Clotting of milk   Heating milk
The various forms in which milk can be purchased
Comparison of nutritive content of milks   *Experiments*

8   MILK PRODUCTS   93

Cream   *Experiment*   Butter   *Experiment*   Cheese   Yogurt
Ice cream

9   EGGS   99

Composition of an egg   Nutrient content
Changes which occur during storage   Methods used to preserve eggs
Uses of eggs in cookery   Effect of various agents on egg white foam
Experiments with eggs

10   MEAT, POULTRY AND FISH   112

The structure of meat   Post mortem changes   The cooking of meat
Nutritional value of meat
Fish   Nutritional value of fish   *Practical work on meat and fish*

11 **CEREALS** 121

Nutritional value of common cereals   Rice
Experimental cooking of rice   Maize   Barley   Oats   Rye
Practical work   Millets   Wheat   Strong and weak wheats
The milling of wheat   The bleaching of flour   Improving flour
Extraction rates of flour   Bread   Baking technology
Experimental breadmaking

12 **STARCHES** 134

Raising agents   *Experiments*   Starches
The extraction of starch from wheat   Chemical structure of starch
Use of starch in the diet   Uses of starch in cookery
Experimental study of starches

13 **SUGARS** 138

Monosaccharides   Disaccharides   Extraction of sugar from the cane
Refining of raw sugar   Properties of sucrose   Uses of sucrose in cookery
Sugar boiling   *Experiments*

14 **FATS AND OILS** 145

Properties of fats and oils   Commercial sources of fat products
The manufacture of margarine   Hydrogenation   Cooking fats
Uses of fats in cooking   *Experiments*

15 **VEGETABLES AND FRUITS** 150

The nutritional value of some common vegetables   The potato
Fruits   Nutritional value of some common fruits
Nutritional value of some common nuts
The structure of fruits and vegetables
Effect of cooking on the structure of plant cells   Plant pigments
Browning reactions   Prevention of browning
Experimental work on fruits and vegetables

Table: Recommended Daily Intakes of Energy and Nutrients for the UK (1969)   **164**

Index   **170**

Acknowledgment

Diagrams of cereals, sugar cane and sugar beet have been based on drawings by Barbara Nicholson from *The Oxford Book of Food Plants* by S. G. Harrison, G. B. Masefield and M. Wallis and are reproduced by permission of the publishers, The Clarendon Press, Oxford.

Many of the figures for the nutrient content of foods have been obtained from *The Composition of Foods* by R. A. McCance and E. M. Widdowson, by kind permission of Her Majesty's Stationary Office.

My grateful thanks are due to Gillian Calver (née Burnett) who undertook the tedious task of checking the text.

Margaret Knight
1976

Preface

This book is designed to help the teacher to instruct students in the subjects of Nutrition and Food Science. It is suitable for the A level Home Economics syllabus, O level Food and Nutrition, Royal Society of Health Nutrition Certificate and Diploma, City and Guilds Home Economics and Catering courses, for Catering and Domestic Science Colleges and indeed anyone interested in food. Many students of Nutrition and Food Science will also find this book invaluable.

The Nutrition section has been kept brief as there are many books dealing with this subject. The Food Science section has been strengthened with a wide range of experiments.

When teaching Nutrition one has to remember that people eat foods rather than nutrients and therefore it is important to relate nutrients to their food sources in a practical way. A set of food tables per student is a necessity. Students should constantly be looking up the energy value, protein, calcium, iron and vitamin C values (and often other nutrients) of common foods so that they become familiar with the food value of the foods they eat. Daily allowances of the common nutrients should be shown to the students in terms of foods they might eat in a day. This is especially important for iron where there may be a shortage. It is interesting to include foods from other countries so that students can appreciate how it can be difficult to obtain, for example, the daily protein allowance in a country where fish, meat and dairy produce are in short supply. The food tables given in *The Composition of Tropical Foods* by B S Platt (HMSO 1945) are useful here.

Students must learn weights of typical portions of food eaten. This can be done by having a pair of scales available and weighing foods that are about to be eaten at a meal. Once this has been carried out a few times, the weight of such foods as an egg, a rasher of bacon, a slice of bread, an apple, a portion of meat and portions of potatoes, other vegetables, and fruit will be familiar to the student. Knowing the weights of typical portions of food it is then possible to assess the value of a person's diet even though the foods have not been weighed.

Preface

A good exercise using food tables is to get the students to weigh every food that they eat for three days and then to work out their average daily Calorie (or megajoule), protein, fat, calcium, iron, vitamin A, C and D intake.

There is a wide range of Nutrition films which are extremely useful when used in conjunction with teaching. See page 165.

Digestion is a vital part of the Nutrition syllabus and is often little understood. A life size anatomical model is an aid in showing the position of the organs in the alimentary canal and there are several good films on the subject. Experiments illustrating enzyme action are important.

Food Science is a subject which cannot be taught without a large quantity of practical work. At least half of each class should be devoted to practical work and visits to food manufacturers and a flour mill help to increase the students' knowledge.

A few good quality microscopes are essential so that the students can see the detailed structure of such things as starch grains, meat fibres and emulsions. Most of the experiments can be made in a laboratory using simple equipment, but some of the experiments require an oven and therefore will have to be done in a kitchen.

There are often many additional variations not mentioned in this book which can be made to the experiments if the class is large. The number of experiments which are suitable for any given class will have to be selected carefully by the teacher, according to class size, age group of students, equipment and time available. If the class is large, and time or equipment limited, many experiments can be shown to the class as demonstrations. Each student should have a notebook and write up each experiment with a Method, Results and Conclusion. They should note down the results obtained by their fellow students in the variants.

People engaged in preparing food are usually too busy trying to achieve a product of a high standard to have time to think about what function individual ingredients have, but by the time they have worked through these experiments there should be a greater understanding of this. If a poor result is obtained in food preparation it should be easier to ascertain what was at fault.

1
Introduction to Nutrition and Food Science

In order to have some understanding of food science it is necessary to comprehend the chemical composition of food and also the properties exhibited by the various nutrients.

Firstly, all food is made up of minute particles called *atoms*.

DEFINITION OF AN ATOM

An atom is the smallest part of a substance which can take part in a chemical reaction. Atoms tend to be attracted to other atoms. Where there is a union of two or more atoms a *molecule* is formed.

Atoms are usually represented diagrammatically as spheres. A molecule of water is shown thus:

(H) + (H) + (O) ⟶ (O/H H)

2 atoms of hydrogen + 1 atom of oxygen = 1 molecule of water.
A molecule of carbon dioxide would be:
1 atom of carbon + 2 atoms of oxygen = 1 molecule of carbon dioxide.

(C) + (O) + (O) ⟶ (C/O O)

A molecule of sodium chloride (common salt) is:

(Na) + (Cl) ⟶ (Na)(Cl)

1 atom of sodium + 1 atom of chlorine = 1 molecule of sodium chloride.
Foods are made up from molecules of water, protein, fat, carbo-

hydrate, vitamins and minerals; their structure will be shown later.

Atoms of the same type existing together form *elements*.

DEFINITION OF AN ELEMENT

An element is a simple substance consisting of only one type of atom. Thus atoms in an element are all identical but they are very different from the atoms in any other element. Elements are divided into two categories — metals and non-metals.

Examples of elements which are metals

Copper, iron, lead, mercury, sodium, potassium, zinc, calcium aluminium and tin.

Examples of elements which are non-metals

Carbon, sulphur, phosphorus, oxygen, nitrogen, hydrogen and iodine.

Carbon, hydrogen and oxygen are important in the study of foods as they are present in proteins, fats and carbohydrates.

Elements combine together to form *compounds*.

DEFINITION OF A COMPOUND

A compound is a combination of two or more elements which are chemically united. A compound always has a definite 'recipe', thus water contains one atom of the element oxygen for every two atoms of the element hydrogen that are present. Compounds can only be split into their constituent elements by chemical means.

1 molecule of the compound sucrose (cane sugar) contains 12 atoms of carbon, 22 atoms of hydrogen and 11 atoms of oxygen.

12 atoms of carbon + 22 atoms of hydrogen + 11 atoms of oxygen =
1 molecule of the compound sucrose

$$12\,C + 22\,H + 11\,O = C_{12}H_{22}O_{11}$$

If there are only 21 atoms of hydrogen available the compound sucrose cannot be made. A sample of a compound will normally consist of vast numbers of molecules.

Examples of compounds

Sodium chloride, copper sulphate, hydrochloric acid, water, calcium carbonate, sodium bicarbonate and sulphur dioxide.

Examples of compounds present in foods

Amino acids, glycerol, fatty acids, starches, sugars, pectin and cellulose.

MIXTURES

If elements and compounds are mixed together in varying proportions, mixtures are made. Mixtures have no fixed composition and they can be separated into their constituents by physical means.

Examples of mixtures

Air is a typical mixture as its composition varies from one area to another. Milk is a mixture as samples of milk, even from the same cow, can vary in composition according to the time of year, the diet eaten, etc.

PRACTICAL WORK

1   Set out a display of metals and non-metals on watch glasses. Include iron, copper, carbon, phosphorus, calcium, sodium, magnesium, iodine and potassium which are important in nutrition.
2   Set out a display of compounds on watch glasses. Include sugar, starch, water, sodium chloride and glycerol which are nutrients used by the body.

EXPERIMENTS

1   *Experiment to show that the compound sucrose can be split by chemical means*
Apparatus
   1 evaporating dish on an asbestos mat
   1 pipette
Reagents
   Sucrose (cane sugar)
   Concentrated sulphuric acid

Cover the bottom of the evaporating dish with sucrose. Add a few drops of water to the sucrose (this helps to speed up the reaction) and then add concentrated sulphuric acid drop by drop with a pipette. Place in a fume cupboard.
Results
Dense fumes are evolved and the sucrose turns black.
Explanation
Concentrated sulphuric acid is a powerful dehydrating agent, ie it has an affinity for water. Sucrose consists of carbon and water, the acid removes the water and leaves the black charcoal.

$$C_{12}H_{22}O_{11} - 11\,H_2O = 12\,C$$
$$\text{Sucrose} \qquad \text{Water} \quad \text{Carbon}$$

2   *Experiment to show that a mixture of sugar and sand can be separated by physical means*
Apparatus

1 beaker	Evaporating dish
Glass stirring rod	Bunsen burner
Glass filter funnel	Tripod, gauze
Filter paper	

Introduction to Nutrition and Food Science

Materials
A mixture of sugar and sand
Method
Place a small quantity of the mixture in a beaker and add some water. Stir and warm to dissolve the sugar. Filter the mixture through a filter paper placed in a glass funnel into an evaporating dish. Heat the liquid in the evaporating dish to dryness.

Results
The sand is retained on the filter paper and the sugar is in the evaporating dish.

Explanation
Sugar particles are soluble in water and these molecules pass through the filter paper. Sand particles are not soluble in water and are too large to pass through the filter paper. Thus this mixture can be separated into its components by physical means.

Chemical and physical changes occurring in food preparation
There are two types of changes which occur in food preparation:
1 Physical changes
2 Chemical changes

Physical changes	Chemical changes
1 The conversion of water into ice and steam. If the conditions are reversed the reaction reverses and the original substance is reformed. Ice, water and steam are chemically the same but their physical state is different. $$\text{ICE} \underset{\text{Cool}}{\overset{\text{Heat}}{\rightleftarrows}} \text{WATER} \underset{\text{Cool}}{\overset{\text{Heat}}{\rightleftarrows}} \text{STEAM}$$ 2 Melting of wax $$\text{Solid wax} \underset{\text{Cool}}{\overset{\text{Heat}}{\rightleftarrows}} \text{Liquid wax}$$	1 Combustion. If a piece of wood or paper is burnt gases are formed and ash which are new chemicals. If conditions are reversed the original substances cannot be obtained. $$\text{WOOD} \xrightarrow{\text{Combustion}} \text{ASH} + \text{GASES}$$ 2 Formation of rust. Once rust is formed on iron a new chemical is formed and conditions cannot be reversed.

Osmosis

Examples of chemical and physical changes taking place in food preparation

Physical changes	*Chemical changes*
Preparation of a jelly using gelatine. Jelly can be heated to liquefy it and cooled to make it solid. Preparation of a salad dressing — Oil and vinegar are shaken together. When allowed to stand, the oil forms a layer on the top and can be separated from the vinegar.	Making of toast. Starch is converted into dextrin Cooking an egg. Gelatinisation of starch. Browning of fruit. Cooking of meat, fish and poultry. Cooking of vegetables. In all these examples reactions take place which cannot be reversed on reversing the conditions. Most of these examples will be dealt with more fully later on in the book.

OSMOSIS

This is the process during which water molecules move from an area of low solute concentration to an area of high solute concentration through a semi-permeable membrane until concentrations are equal on both sides of the membrane.

A semi-permeable membrane is one which contains pores of a size which allow the water molecules to pass through them but prevents the passage of the larger solute molecules. Cell walls are examples of semi-permeable membranes. In the diagram shown on the following page, the water molecules move mainly from the left to the right through the membrane until the concentrations are equal on both sides of the membrane. Some water molecules can move from right to left but these will be swamped by the large number of water molecules moving in the opposite direction.

Osmosis occurs in food preparation when for example there is a cell wall separating solutions of different osmotic pressures. If a prune is soaked in water it swells. This is because the osmotic pressure inside the prune is greater than the osmotic pressure of the water. Water molecules move through the skin and swell the prune. Similarly when fruit is bottled, if the syrup is weak water moves into the fruit or if the syrup is too strong water moves out of the fruit and it shrinks.

Diagram to illustrate osmosis taking place between two sugar solutions separated by a semi-permeable membrane

Weak sugar solution | Strong sugar solution

o Water molecules
O Sugar molecules
Semi-permeable membrane

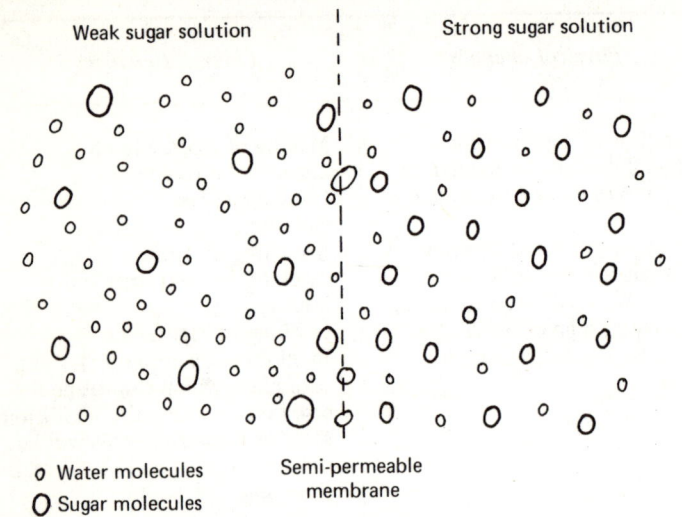

Experiments with osmosis
1 Soak a prune in water to show swelling due to osmosis.
2 Take 2 potatoes, peel them, cut a well in each and cut the rounded end from each so the potatoes will stand. Place the first potato in a bowl and surround it with water. Put salt solution in the well. Place the second potato in another bowl and surround it with salt solution and put water in the well. Note height of liquid in the well in each case. Leave for several hours and then note the height of the liquid in each well.

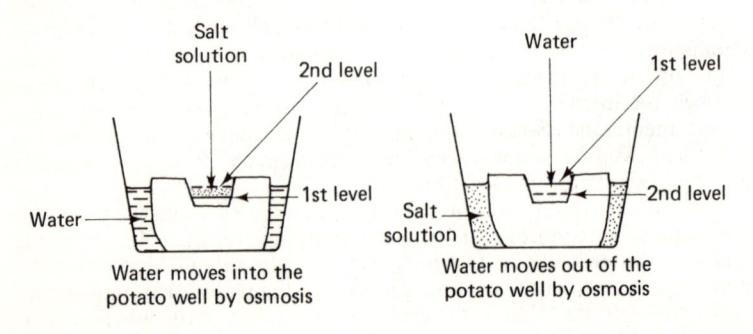

Water moves into the potato well by osmosis

Water moves out of the potato well by osmosis

Diffusion

3 Place 2 eggs in some dilute hydrochloric acid overnight to dissolve away the shell. The shell membrane remains intact. Put one of the eggs in a beaker containing concentrated salt solution and one egg in dilute salt solution.

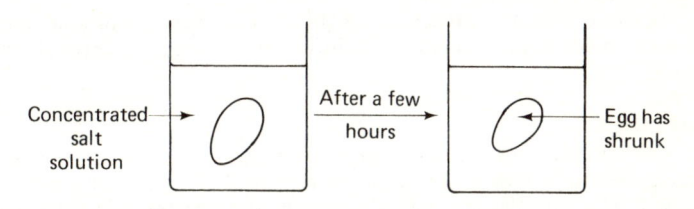

The osmotic pressure of the salt solution is greater than that of the egg so water moves out of the egg. The egg shell membrane is a semipermeable membrane.

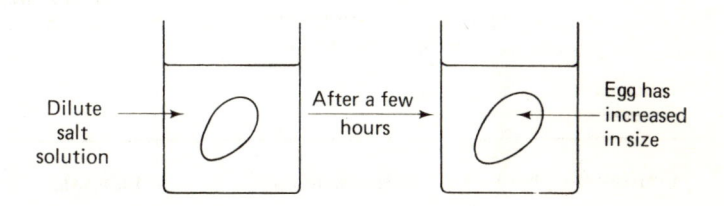

The osmotic pressure of the egg is greater than that of the dilute salt solution so water molecules move into the egg.

DIFFUSION

This is the process in which the molecules move from a region of high concentration to a region of lower concentration until the concentrations are equal.

Diffusion of gases can be shown if a coloured gas is released in an enclosed area, gradually the gas spreads throughout the area until the colour is the same throughout the area and the concentration of the gas will also be the same throughout provided the gas has the same density as the atmosphere. Diffusion in solids and liquids can be seen if a soluble coloured crystal is put in a beaker of water. The colour throughout the beaker gradually becomes the same as the molecules of solute move from a region of high concentration to a region of low concentration.

Diffusion is constantly occurring in food preparation where the tendency is for solute molecules to move until concentrations are equal throughout the product.

SOLUTIONS

Many substances dissolve in liquids to form solutions. A solution is clear and homogeneous throughout. Many foods when cooked in water lose some water soluble vitamins and minerals in the cooking water. The cooking water then becomes a solution.

The solid (solute) particles in a solution are very small and cannot be seen under a microscope. A solution passes straight through filter paper.

COLLOIDS

When water is mixed with large molecules, eg those of protein or starch, the molecules do not dissolve to form a solution but a colloid is formed. The particles in a colloidal system will pass through filter paper but will be retained by parchment paper which has smaller pores than filter paper.

In a colloidal solution there are two distinct phases, the solid molecules are called the *disperse phase* and the liquid is called the *continuous phase*. There are many different types of colloidal systems, the disperse phase and the continuous phase can be solids, liquids or gases. Many foods exist in the colloidal stage, eg

Continuous phase	Disperse phase	Examples
Liquid	Gas	Foams, eg egg white foam and whipped cream
Liquid	Liquid	Emulsions, eg milk, mayonnaise, egg yolk, salad dressing
Liquid	Solid	Starch in water, proteins in water
Solid	Gas	Marshmallow, meringues
Solid	Liquid	Jelly. Solid emulsions, eg butter and margarine

EMULSIONS
Emulsions are formed when two immiscible liquids come together. The best example is a mixture of oil and water, when such a mixture is shaken up the oil splits into droplets forming an emulsion. On standing the oil droplets join together and the oil forms a layer on top of the water. Such emulsions are said to be temporary. An emulsifying agent needs to be present to form a permanent emulsion. An example of a permanent emulsion is mayonnaise, the emulsifying agent is lecithin in egg yolk. Mayonnaise is an oil in water emulsion as the oil droplets are dispersed in the liquid vinegar. Butter is a water in oil emulsion as the water droplets are dispersed in the continuous phase, the fat. The milk proteins act as emulsifying agents.

Gravies and sauces are emulsions which are stabilised with flour. Flour is an inefficient emulsifying agent so there should be a high percentage of water and a low percentage of oil present. If there is too much oil present large globules will form.

SUSPENSIONS
Suspensions are mixtures of solids and liquids, they contain large particles which are insoluble and visible to the naked eye. The particles are retained by filter and parchment paper. If the mixture is left undisturbed the solid particles gradually settle to the bottom of the suspension leaving the liquid above them.

Nutrients are present in foods generally in the following physical states:
Sugars – form solutions.
Starches – form suspensions in cold water and a colloidal gel in hot water.
Fats – form emulsions.
Proteins are present as colloids.
Vitamins and minerals are present in solutions.

Experiment to compare the effectiveness of various substances as emulsifying agents
1   Place 5 ml of oil into each of 6 test tubes.
2   Add 2 ml of one of the following solutions to each – 50% egg solution, 50% egg yolk solution, vinegar, 1% sugar solution, 1% starch solution and 1% gelatine solution.
   Shake each tube for 2 minutes.
3   Note type of emulsion formed in each tube.
   Which solution is the most effective emulsifying agent?

Acidity and alkalinity of food
The degree of acidity or alkalinity a food possesses can be expressed on the pH Scale. This scale was set up so that an exact value of

acidity or alkalinity could be obtained. Water being a neutral substance is found in the middle of the scale and given a pH of 7.

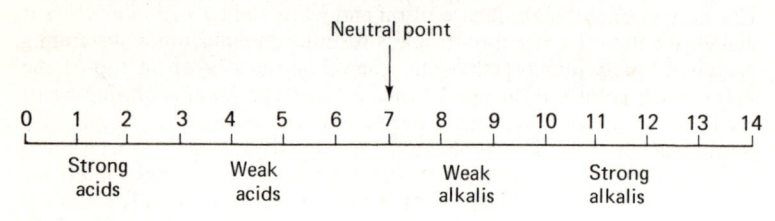

```
                    Neutral point
                         |
                         ↓
 0   1   2   3   4   5   6   7   8   9   10   11   12   13   14
 └───┴───┴───┴───┴───┴───┴───┴───┴───┴────┴────┴────┴────┴────┘
        Strong         Weak              Weak          Strong
        acids          acids             alkalis       alkalis
```

The pH numbers indicate the concentration of hydrogen ions in logarithmic numbers.

If a substance has a low pH it will be very acid, if it has a value of 5 or 6 it will be only slightly acidic. If a substance has a pH of 8 or 9 it is weakly alkaline and a pH of 12 or 13 will indicate a strong alkaline.

Strong acid foods
  Lemons, vinegar, rhubarb and grapefruit
Medium acid foods
  Pears, bananas, carrots and tomatoes
Weakly acidic foods
  Milk, butter, meat and most vegetables
Alkaline foods
  There are few foods which are alkaline. Egg white and some products made with flour are weak alkalis.

The pH of a food can be measured using pH paper, Universal Indicator or a pH meter. A litmus test will only indicate whether the food is acid or alkaline. The pH value of a food affects many of the reactions which take place in cooking. Vitamin C is preserved much more effectively in acid foods than in alkaline foods. The addition of bicarbonate of soda to the cooking water of green vegetables such as cabbage speeds up the destruction of vitamin C. Acid foods are generally easier to preserve than alkaline or neutral foods as many bacteria do not survive at low pHs. The colour of many vegetable and fruit pigments varies according to the pH of the cooking water.

When milk is fresh its pH is about 6.6 as it is kept the lactose (milk sugar) is converted into lactic acid. Between pH 4.5 and 5.0 milk will turn sour and the protein will coagulate. If an acid food such as lemon juice is added to milk this decreases the pH and curdling occurs.

PRACTICAL WORK

Measure the pH of the following foods using pH paper, Universal Indicator or a pH meter: lemon juice, vinegar, egg yolk, egg white, fish, beef, milk, butter, cream, bread, etc.

The solid foods should be ground with a little distilled water before the pH can be ascertained.

2 Digestion and Absorption

The most important physiological function of the body for the student studying food to understand is the process of digestion.

Diagram to show the organs of the human alimentary canal

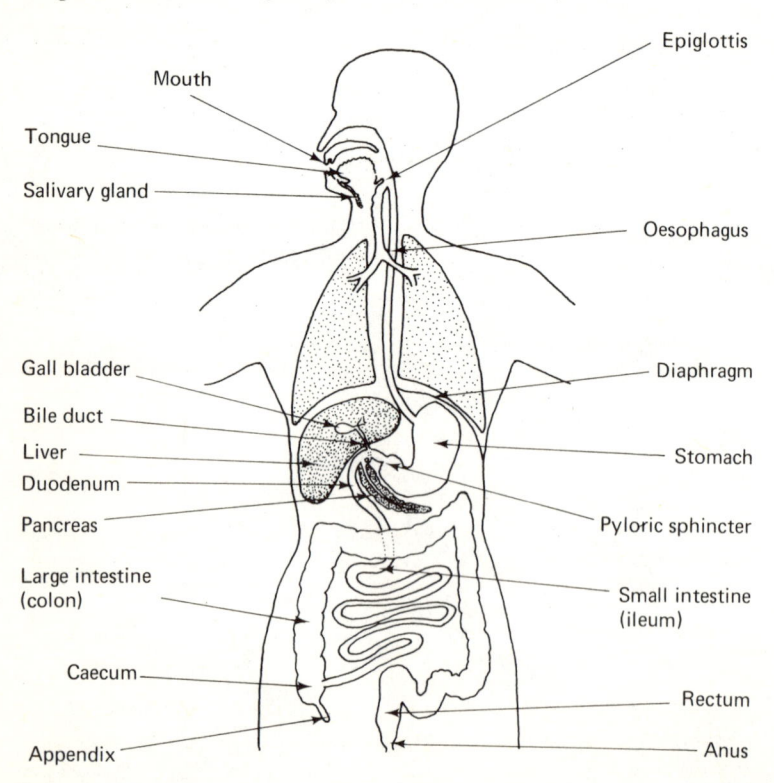

DIGESTION
Digestion is the process in which foods are broken down into simple soluble substances which can be absorbed mainly in the small intestine.

The organs concerned with digestion are the mouth, pharynx, oesophagus, stomach, and the intestines. The liver, gall bladder and the pancreas are accessory organs which aid digestion.

Digestion in the mouth
The sight, smell, thought and taste of food causes the 3 pairs of salivary glands in the mouth to secrete saliva. Saliva is a colourless fluid with a pH of 6.2 − 7.4, it contains mucin, inorganic salts and the enzyme amylase which splits starch into the disaccharide maltose. When food is in the mouth it is chewed and mixed with saliva and in the act of deglutition it passes down the oesophagus to the stomach by peristalsic waves. The food is called *bolus* at this stage.

Diagrams to show peristalsic movements

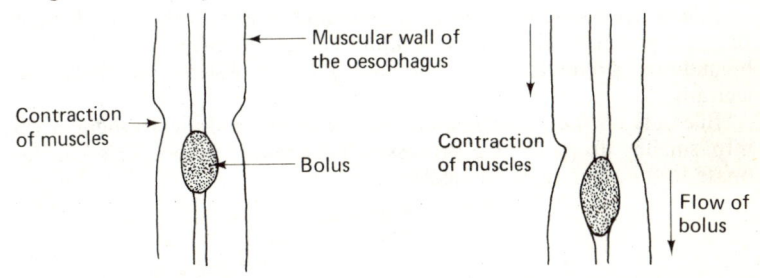

Digestion in the stomach
The muscles in the stomach contract and relax mixing the bolus with the gastric juice. The gastric juice is secreted by glands in the wall of the stomach. It is secreted in response to the presence of food in the stomach and the thought, smell and taste of food. The amount of gastric juice secreted is affected by the type of food that is eaten; protein foods produce the greatest stimulus to gastric secretion.

Content of gastric juice
1   Mucin, this makes the gastric juice thick and opalescent.
2   Intrinsic factor which aids the absorption of vitamin B 12.
3   Electrolytes.
4   Hydrochloric acid. The pH of pure gastric juice is 1.2.
5   Pepsinogen which is converted into pepsin in the presence of hydrochloric acid.
6   Rennin is an enzyme present in the gastric juice of infants which clots milk.

Digestion and Absorption

Functions of gastric juice and the stomach
1   Carries on the mixing of food by muscular contractions.
2   Hydrochloric acid has a bacteriostatic action.
3   The high acid concentration inactivates amylase in the saliva.
4   Some sucrose may be hydrolysed by hydrochloric acid into glucose and fructose.
5   Pepsin converts proteins into proteoses and peptones.
6   Some water, alcohol and certain drugs are absorbed in the stomach.

The food which is now called *chyme* passes into the duodenum through the pyloric sphincter partly due to peristaltic waves and partly because of a build up of pressure in the stomach. Gastric emptying is also affected by the composition of the food; if fat is present gastric emptying is slowed up.

Digestion in the small intestine
Once the chyme is in the small intestine, bile is released from the gall bladder and passes down the bile duct and is poured on to the food in the duodenum.

Bile is synthesised in the liver cells and stored in the gall bladder. Bile is a greenish-yellow viscous liquid containing pigments (which are breakdown products of haemoglobin), electrolytes, bile salts and lecithin.

Bile acts on the globules of fat in the chyme and breaks them down into smaller droplets in a process called emulsification. This enables lipase to function more efficiently.

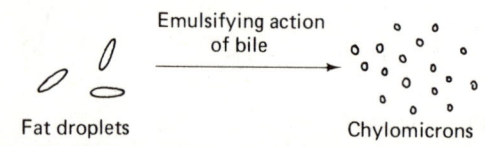

Fat droplets → Emulsifying action of bile → Chylomicrons

Diagram to show the position of the liver and gall bladder

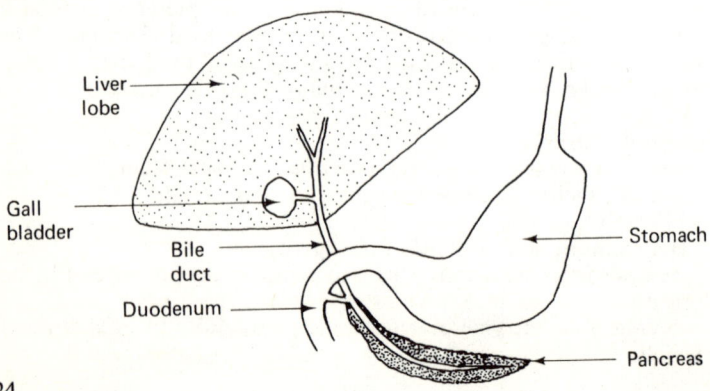

(Labels: Liver lobe, Gall bladder, Bile duct, Duodenum, Stomach, Pancreas)

Digestion

Pancreatic juices are poured on to the food when it is in the small intestine.

Content of the pancreatic juices
1. Trypsinogen which is converted into its active form trypsin by enterokinase. Trypsin acts on proteoses and peptones and breaks them down into shorter chain peptides.
2. Chymotrypsinogen is converted into its active form chymotrypsin by trypsin. The chymotrypsin also breaks down proteoses and peptones into shorter chain peptides.
3. Amylase, which acts on starch breaking it down to maltose.
4. Lipase, which acts on the emulsified fats and converts them to fatty acids and glycerol.

```
    H                                H
    |                                |
H — C — OCO Fatty acid 1       H — C — OH        Fatty acid 1
    |                 Lipase        |
H — C — OCO Fatty acid 2   →   H — C — OH    +   Fatty acid 2
    |                                |
H — C — OCO Fatty acid 3       H — C — OH        Fatty acid 3
    |                                |
    H                                H

  Triglyceride                    Glycerol          3 Fatty acids
```

This reaction can be represented diagramatically thus:

```
  ┌─────                        ┌─────
  │                             │
  │           Lipase            │                   ─────
  │          ─────→             │           +
  │                             │                   ─────
  └─────                        │
                                └─────              ─────
```

5. Many electrolytes are present. The bicarbonate concentration is especially high. The pH of the pancreatic juice is 8.6.

The pancreas also produces the hormone insulin which circulates in the blood system and controls blood glucose levels.

Glands in the wall of the small intestine are stimulated to produce intestinal juices when the food is present in the duodenum.

Content of the intestinal juices
1. Peptidases, which split short chain peptides into amino acids.
2. Sucrase, which splits sucrose into glucose and fructose.
3. Lactase which splits lactose into glucose and galactose.
4. Maltase which splits maltose into two molecules of glucose.

Digestion and Absorption

5   Lipase which splits fat into glycerol and fatty acids.

At this stage the three main classes of nutrients to be digested, ie the proteins, fats and carbohydrates, have been split into simple units which are ready for absorption. The proteins are in the form of amino acids, the fats have been reduced to glycerol and fatty acids and the carbohydrates into the simple sugars, glucose, galactose and fructose.

Absorption of the nutrients in the small intestine
Diagrammatic representation of a vertical section through the villi in the small intestine

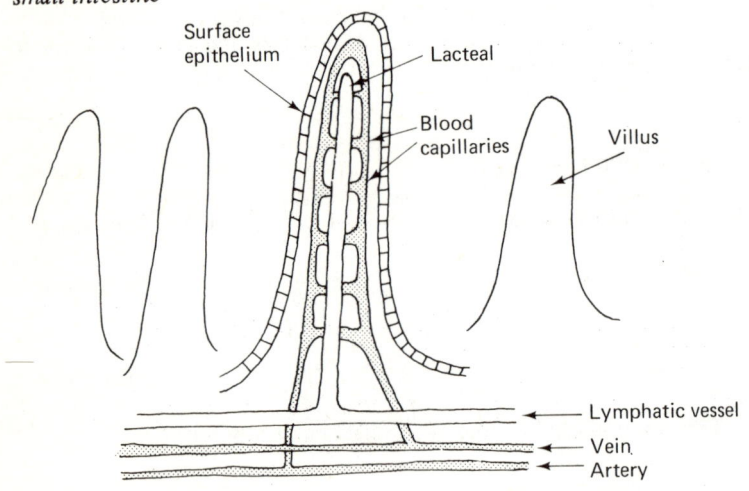

Surface epithelium
Lacteal
Blood capillaries
Villus
Lymphatic vessel
Vein
Artery

Absorption and utilisation of sugars

Simple sugars (glucose, fructose and galactose)

Absorbed by diffusion in the small intestine

Travel to the liver in the hepatic portal vein

Used as an energy source | Converted into glycogen | Stored as fat in adipose tissue

The sugars in the small intestine pass by diffusion into the blood vessels of the villi. The different sugars are absorbed at varying speeds.

Galactose is absorbed the quickest, then glucose and then fructose. The sugars are carried to the liver in the hepatic portal vein. These sugars may be used for energy or they are converted into glycogen and stored in the liver and muscles. Some sugar can be converted into fat and stored in the adipose tissue.

Absorption and utilisation of fats

Most of the fatty acids and the glycerol combine together to form triglycerides as they diffuse into the cells of the villi. The recombined fats then pass into the lacteals. The fats travel from the lacteals in the lymphatic system to the great veins in the neck where they are poured out into the general circulation.

This fat can then be used as a source of energy, supplying 9 Calories per gramme, or it is stored in fat depots. The fat in the fat depots can be mobilised and used as a source of energy. Unfortunately this process is not very efficient in most people as those who have been on a slimming diet will have experienced. As soon as they cut down their food intake they find that the conversion of fat into energy is slow so they experience a feeling of weakness. Some fat passes into the capillaries of the villi and travels direct to the liver where it can be used as energy source or for the synthesis of lipid compounds.

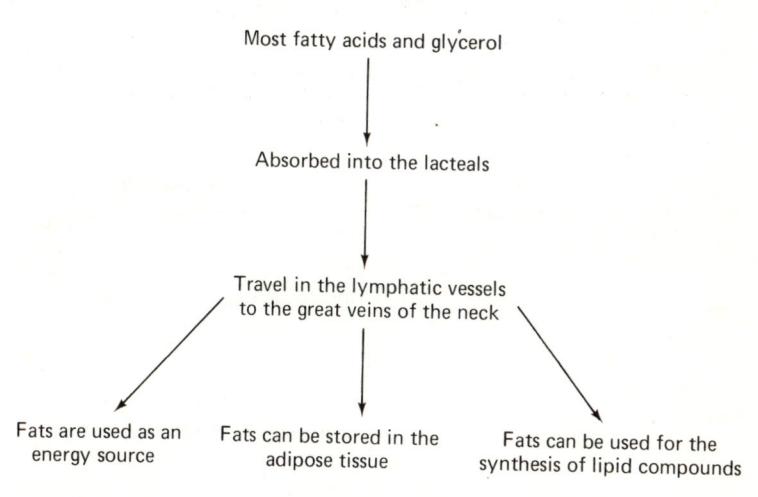

Most fatty acids and glycerol
↓
Absorbed into the lacteals
↓
Travel in the lymphatic vessels to the great veins of the neck
↙ ↓ ↘
Fats are used as an energy source | Fats can be stored in the adipose tissue | Fats can be used for the synthesis of lipid compounds

Absorption and utilisation of proteins

The amino acids in the small intestine diffuse into the blood vessels in the villi and travel in the hepatic portal vessel to the liver. The most important use of amino acids in the body is for the synthesis of proteins. The amino acids circulate in the blood stream and are absorbed by the cells and used for protein synthesis.

If available supplies of fat and carbohydrate have been used up then some amino acids are used as a source of energy. The amino acids to be used for energy are first broken down in a process called deamination which takes place in the liver. The nitrogen part of the amino acid is converted to ammonia and the non-nitrogenous part goes through a series of complex reactions and finally yields energy. Excess amino acids can be converted into fat and stored.

The ammonia, being toxic, has to be converted into a compound which is less toxic, ie urea. The ammonia passes through what is known as the urea cycle in the liver. The urea then passes into the general circulation, and is filtered off by the kidneys and together with water, mineral salts, etc, forms urine.

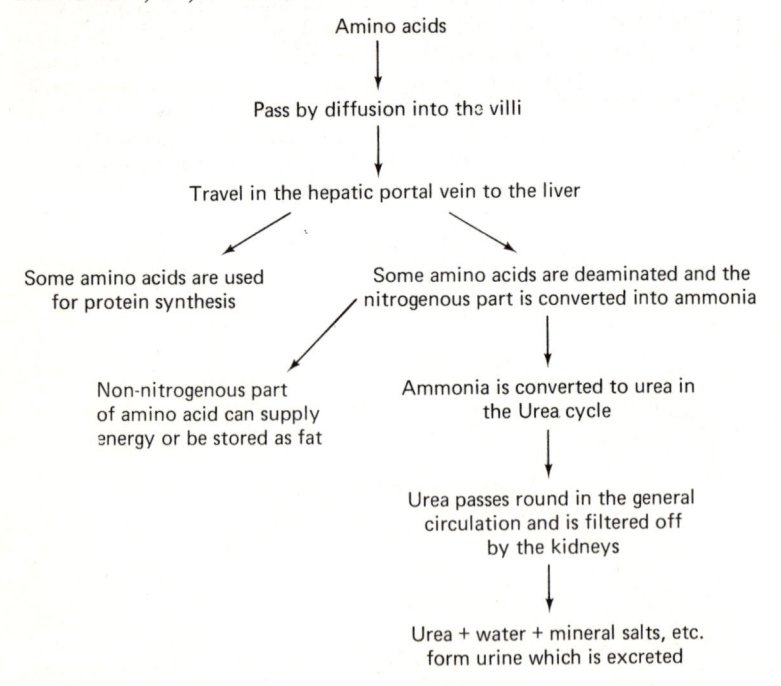

Amino acids
↓
Pass by diffusion into the villi
↓
Travel in the hepatic portal vein to the liver
↙ ↘
Some amino acids are used for protein synthesis

Some amino acids are deaminated and the nitrogenous part is converted into ammonia
↓
Non-nitrogenous part of amino acid can supply energy or be stored as fat

Ammonia is converted to urea in the Urea cycle
↓
Urea passes round in the general circulation and is filtered off by the kidneys
↓
Urea + water + mineral salts, etc. form urine which is excreted

Absorption of vitamins, minerals and water

The mineral salts diffuse into the villi and travel in the hepatic portal vein to the liver from whence they go in the blood stream to the cells of the body that require them. Excess mineral salts are excreted. Absorption of water soluble vitamins takes place rapidly by diffusion

Practical Work

and most of the fat soluble vitamins are absorbed with the fat. Some water is absorbed by osmosis in the stomach but most is absorbed in the small intestine.

The formation of faeces

The food which has not been digested and absorbed passes into the large intestine. In the large intestine more water is absorbed from the food residue making the mass more solid. The faeces are expelled from the rectum via the anus. The faeces contain cellulose, bacteria, dead cells, bile pigments, mucous and salts.

PRACTICAL WORK ON DIGESTION

1   Observe slides of the alimentary canal under the microscope, ie sections of the small intestine to show the villi and lacteals, sections of the stomach to show the glands producing gastric juice, sections of the pancreas to show regions producing the pancreatic juice and region secreting insulin.

2   Location of areas of tongue responsive to 4 basic tastes. The taste buds in the tongue are responsive to 4 tastes, sweet, sour, salt and bitter and they are located in certain areas of the tongue.
Method
   Dip a moist glass rod into sugar and place on the front, back and sides of the tongue. Note area where the sensation of sweetness is received. Repeat with salt, quinine which is bitter and alum which is sour.

EXPERIMENTS

1   **Experiment to demonstrate the action of amylase in the saliva**
Apparatus
   One white tile
   One teat pipette
   10 ml pipette
   3 ml pipette
   One thermometer
   Waterbath
   Four test tubes in rack
Reagents
   Saliva
   Iodine solution
   1% starch solution
Method
   Place small drops of iodine solution in neat rows on a white tile. Take 4 test tubes. Into test tubes 1 and 2 pipette 10 ml of starch solution.

Digestion and Absorption

Into test tube 3 pipette 3 ml of saliva and into test tube 4 pipette 3 ml of saliva which has been thoroughly boiled. Incubate all tubes at 37°C for 5 minutes.

Transfer 3 ml of unboiled saliva into test tube 1, mix and start the stop-watch. At once withdraw 1 drop of the mixture and allow it to fall on 1 drop of the iodine solution. Every half minute withdraw a drop of the starch-saliva mixture and allow it to fall on to a drop of iodine. Continue until there is no colour change when the mixture of starch and saliva comes into contact with the iodine and note the time.

Repeat the experiment with 3 ml of boiled saliva and again note the time taken for the digest to produce no colour change with the iodine.

What effect does boiling have on the saliva?

2 **Experiment to show the action of sucrase in the intestinal juice**
Apparatus
   10 ml pipette
   Three 2 ml pipettes
   Test tubes in rack
   Waterbath
Reagents
   Fehling's solutions
   1% sucrose solution
   Sucrase solution
Method
   Dilute the Fehling's solutions using 1 part of Fehling's solution to 2 parts of water. Pipette 2 ml of this dilution into test tubes A, B, C and D. Prepare 2 digests as follows, into tube 1 pipette 10 ml of 1% sucrose solution and 2 ml of sucrase and into Tube 2 pipette 10 ml of sucrose solution and 2 ml of boiled sucrase. At once withdraw 2 ml from tube 1 and place in tube A and 2 ml from tube 2 and place in tube B. Boil tubes A and B.

Place tubes 1 and 2 in a water bath at 37°C for 10 minutes. Withdraw 2 ml from tube 1 and add to tube C and 2 ml from tube 2 and add to tube D.

Boil tubes C and D and note any colour changes.
Note Sucrose has no effect on Fehling's solution, but when sucrose is split into glucose and fructose by sucrase there is a positive reaction. Glucose and fructose are reducing sugars which reduce Fehling's solution to brick red copper oxide. When sucrase is boiled it is inactivated.

A positive Fehling's test should be obtained for tube C. In tube A the sucrase will not have had time to react.

Absorption

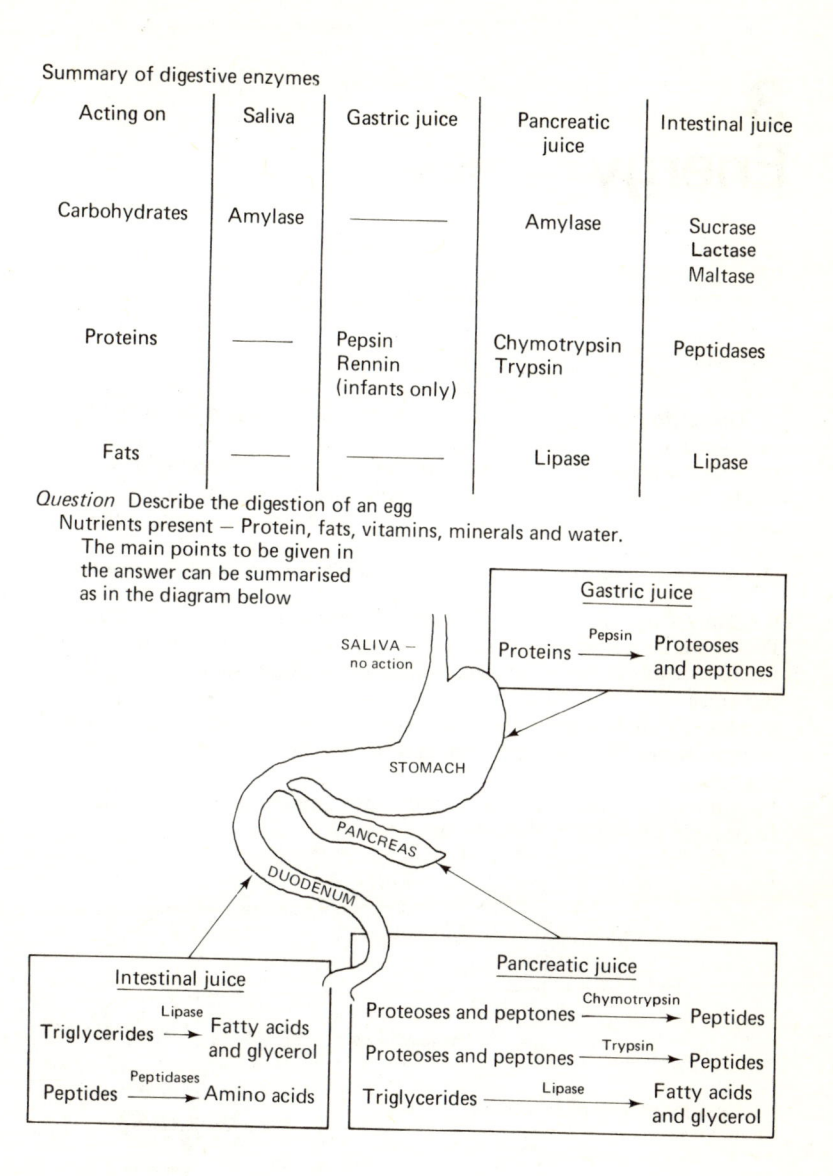

Summary of digestive enzymes

Acting on	Saliva	Gastric juice	Pancreatic juice	Intestinal juice
Carbohydrates	Amylase	—	Amylase	Sucrase Lactase Maltase
Proteins	—	Pepsin Rennin (infants only)	Chymotrypsin Trypsin	Peptidases
Fats	—	—	Lipase	Lipase

Question Describe the digestion of an egg

Nutrients present — Protein, fats, vitamins, minerals and water.
The main points to be given in the answer can be summarised as in the diagram below

Gastric juice

Proteins —Pepsin→ Proteoses and peptones

SALIVA — no action

STOMACH

PANCREAS

DUODENUM

Intestinal juice

Triglycerides —Lipase→ Fatty acids and glycerol

Peptides —Peptidases→ Amino acids

Pancreatic juice

Proteoses and peptones —Chymotrypsin→ Peptides

Proteoses and peptones —Trypsin→ Peptides

Triglycerides —Lipase→ Fatty acids and glycerol

31

3
Energy

The prime source of our energy is the sun which radiates light and heat to the earth. Plants are able to make their own food from the raw materials water, carbon dioxide and energy from the sunlight. Chlorophyll, the green pigment in plants, must also be present. This process is called *photosynthesis*, and can be represented by the following equation.

$$\text{Water + Carbon Dioxide + Energy from Sunlight} \xrightarrow{\text{Chlorophyll}} \text{Sugar + Oxygen}$$

Plants store the sugar in the form of starch in roots, tubers and fruit. Plants are also able to synthesise fats and proteins. This is quite obvious in plants such as the olive tree, the castor oil plant, soya bean plant and nut trees.

Man is unable to make his food from simple raw materials and energy from the sunlight but has to be dependent on plants and animals.

Animals and man eat plants and other animals and oxidise the food to provide themselves with energy.

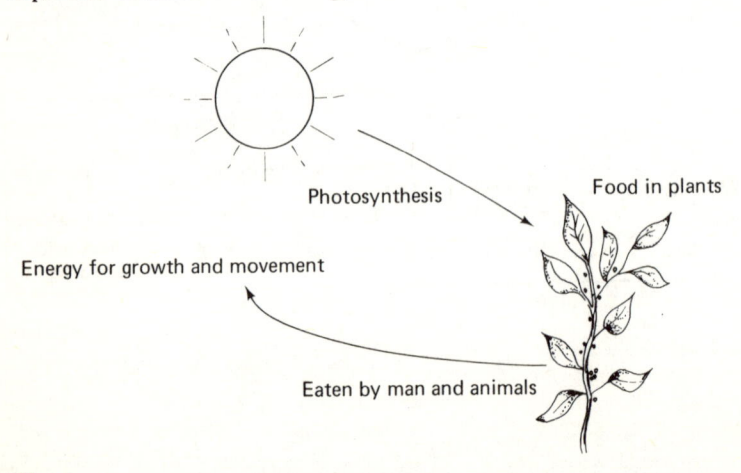

When animals convert plants into their body flesh there is a considerable loss of energy. In view of the general world shortage of food it would seem sensible for man to eat plants to avoid loss of energy. However, animal protein is more valuable to man than plant protein and so it is worth losing some energy to produce it. Also animals are able to convert plant material which is not valuable to man into valuable foods, eg the ruminants are able to convert grass with its high cellulose content into useful food.

ENERGY

Energy can be defined as capacity for doing work. There are many different types of energy, eg mechanical, magnetic, electrical, heat, light and chemical energy. The different forms of energy can often be converted into another form eg electrical energy can be changed into heat energy in an electric fire.

Man obtains his energy from food in the form of chemical energy and he is able to convert this energy into mechanical energy for movement, heartbeat, etc. Unfortunately, the conversion of the chemical energy in food into mechanical energy is only about 25% efficient. The other 75% of the energy is lost as heat energy, some of which is used to maintain the body temperature. If the body temperature is high, the heat energy can be used to evaporate sweat from skin.

The mechanical energy formed in man is produced by internal respiration. In this process energy containing food is oxidised in the cells of the body and energy is released together with carbon dioxide and water. The reactions involved are highly complex, this equation is a simplification of the reactions:

Energy containing food + Oxygen = Energy + Carbon dioxide + Water

Uses of energy in the body

1 Most of the energy is used for the functioning of the organs of the body eg for heart beat, respiratory movements, functioning of the liver and the brain, etc.
2 Movement.
3 Growth.
4 Some energy is stored as energy rich compounds which can be converted into energy when required.

In order to compare the energy producing potential of different foods a unit called the *Calorie* (*kilocalorie*) is used. This Calorie must be written with a capital C to distinguish it from the calorie with a small c which is used in physics. The Calorie is 1000 times larger than the calorie and is defined as the amount of heat required to raise the temperature of 1 kg (1000 g) of water through 1°C.

In the future the Calorie will be superseded by the unit called the *joule*. Joules are used in many branches of science as the unit of energy in the metric system.

Energy

A JOULE

1 joule is the amount of energy needed to accelerate a mass of 1 kg by 1 metre/sec/sec over a distance of 1 metre.

$$1 \text{ calorie} = 4.2 \text{ joules (J)}$$
$$1 \text{ Calorie} = 1000 \text{ calories} = 4{,}200 \text{ J}$$
$$1 \text{ Calorie} = 4.2 \text{ kilojoules (kJ)}$$
$$100 \text{ Calories} = 420 \text{ kJ}$$
$$1000 \text{ Calories} = 4{,}200 \text{ kJ}$$
$$= 4.2 \text{ megajoules (MJ)}$$

Thus an adult male's normal Calorie allowance of 3000 Calories becomes 12.6 MJ.

The energy value of a food can be determined by using an instrument called the *bomb calorimeter*.

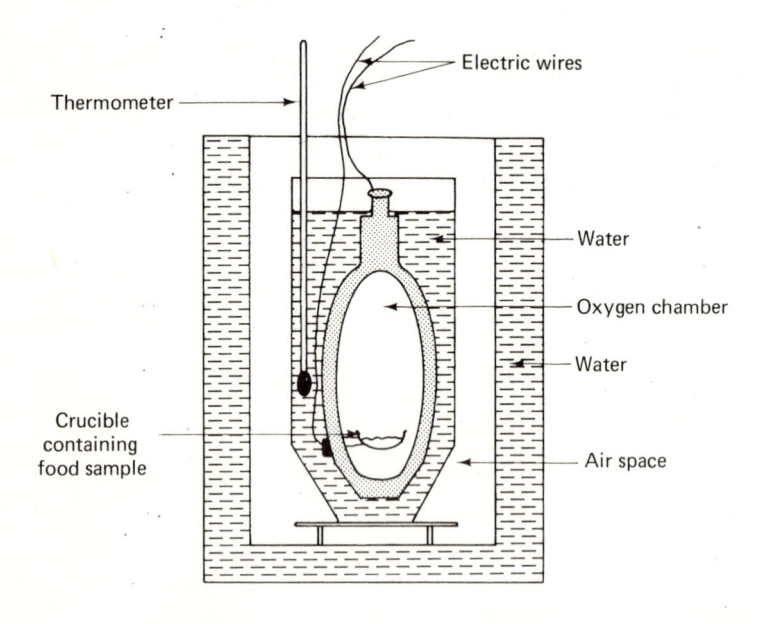

A known weight of food is placed in the crucible in the oxygen chamber. The inner chamber is filled with oxygen and the food sample is ignited electrically. The food sample burns in the oxygen. The heat produced warms the water in the surrounding jacket, the elevation of temperature is read on the thermometer. The greater the energy value of the food the greater will be the rise in temperature of the water. Calculations can then be made to find the calorific value of the food sample.

Energy

The values for the energy producing nutrients are as follows:

	Calories/g	kJ/g
Carbohydrates	4.0	16.8
Fats	9.0	37.8
Protein	4.0	16.8
Alcohol	7.0	29.4

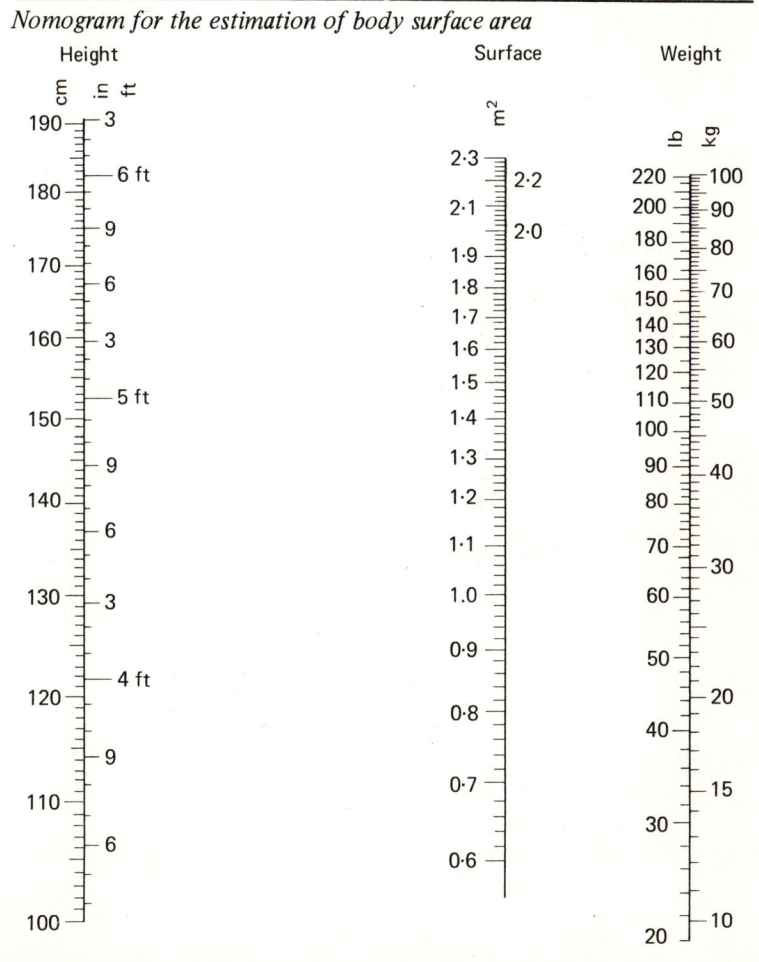

Nomogram for the estimation of body surface area

Energy

Many foods contain two or more nutrients and thus a separate assessment of the energy values has to be made for each food.

THE BASAL METABOLIC RATE
The Basal Metabolic Rate is defined as the rate of energy expenditure when the body is at complete mental and physical rest. It is measured in Calories /sq m of body surface area/hour.

A large proportion of the energy that is produced in the body is used to maintain the Basal Metabolic Rate (BMR).

A typical value for an adult male would be 37 Calories /sq m/hr (155 kJ/sq m/hr). Early measurements on body surface area involved sticking paper all over the body and measuring the area of the paper used. Now there is a convenient way of finding body surface area using the nomogram shown on the previous page. A ruler is placed across the nomogram at points on the scales coinciding with the height and weight of the subject. Where the ruler cuts the area scale this is the figure for the subject's body surface area.

The BMR in Calories/sq m/hour and in kJ/sq m/hour can be found from the following table.

Age yrs	MALES Cals/m^2/hr	MALES kJ/m^2/hr	FEMALES Cals/m^2/hr	FEMALES kJ/m^2/hr
1	53	222	53	222
3	51.3	215	51.2	214
5	49.3	206	48.4	203
7	47.3	198	45.4	190
9	45.2	189	42.8	179
11	43.0	180	42.0	176
13	42.3	177	40.3	169
15	41.8	175	37.9	159
19	39.2	164	35.5	149
20	38.6	162	35.3	148
25	37.5	157	35.2	147
30	36.8	154	35.1	147
40	36.3	152	34.9	146
50	35.8	150	33.9	142
60	34.9	146	32.7	137
70	33.8	141	31.7	133
80	33.0	138	30.9	129

The BMR for the day can be calculated once the body surface area and the BMR in Cals/sq m/hr are known.
Example
What is the BMR of a boy aged 18 years who is 1.8 m tall and weighs 76 kg?
From the nomogram the body surface area is 1.96 sq m.
From the tables the BMR of a boy aged 18 years is 40 Cals/m^2/hr
Therefore the BMR for the whole body surface area will be
40 x 1.96 Cals/hr
= 78.4 Cals/hr
In 24 hours the number of Calories used up in the BMR will be
78.4 x 24 Cals
= 1881.6 Cals
= 7.98 MJ
The BMR is at its maximum during the second year of life and then it gradually declines over the years. The energy used up by the BMR is for respiration, maintenance of heart beat, functioning of the liver, kidneys, brain, etc.

Factors affecting the BMR
1   Body surface area. The greater the body surface area the greater will be the BMR. A tall thin person has a larger surface area than a short fat person.
2   Age. After the age of 2 years the BMR decreases with age.
3   Males have a higher BMR than females.
4   If the body temperature rises by 1°C the BMR goes up by 13%.
5   If the external temperature goes down the BMR rises to help maintain body temperature.
6   During pregnancy the BMR rises
7   Muscular work causes the BMR to rise.
8   The thyroid hormone thyroxine when secreted in excess puts up the BMR. If adrenalin is secreted due to fear or emotion the BMR will rise.

Specific dynamic action of food
This is the stimulation of metabolism due to the intake of food. The SDA can be accounted for by the work of the digestive organs producing their secretions and the metabolism of the liver. Protein foods produce the greatest stimulation to metabolism.

Energy

Energy used in various activities:

	Cals/minute	kJ/minute
Sitting	1.4	5.88
Washing	1.8	7.56
Cooking	2.4	10.08
Bedmaking	7.6	31.92
Writing	1.9	7.98
Cycling	6.6	27.72
Dancing	5.2	21.84
Swimming	9.6	40.32
Tree felling	8.4-12.7	35.28-53.34
Walking	5.3	22.26

Example of daily energy expenditure of an average man

	Calories	MJ
8 hours work at 2.5 Cals/min	1200	5.040
1 hour washing, dressing and undressing at 3 Cals/min	180	0.756
1 hour walking at 5.3 Cals/min	318	1.335
4½ hours sitting at 1.5 Cals/min	405	1.701
1½ hours active recreation at 5.2 Cals/min	468	1.966
8 hours sleep at BMR at 1.04 Cals/min	499.2	2.096
	3070.2	12.894

Energy allowances per day

Boys and girls Years	Calories	Megajoules
0-9	800-2100	3.3-8.8
Boys		
9-12	2500	10.5
12-15	2800	11.7
15-18	3000	12.6
Girls		
9-18	2300	9.6
Males		
18-35	2700-3600	11.3-15.1
	According to occupation	
35-65	2600-3600	10.9-15.1
65+	2350-2100	9.8-8.8
Females		
18-55	2200-2500	9.2-10.5
55-75	2050	8.6
75+	1900	8.0
Pregnancy	2400	10.0
Lactation	2700	11.3

The Calorie intake of adults varies with occupation, eg a coal miner may use up twice as much energy as an office worker.

The Basal Metabolic Rate

The recommended daily intake of Calories decreases with age as the BMR decreases gradually and generally a person becomes more sedentary as they get older.

Weight of food supplying 100 Calories (0.42 MJ) of energy

	g		g
Lard	11	Bread	41
Butter	13	Herring, fried	43
Peanuts	17	Chicken, roast	53
Sweet biscuits	17	Eggs	61
Milk chocolate	17	Baked beans	107
Bacon, back, fried	18	Steamed cod	122
Chocolate cake	20	Potatoes, old, boiled	125
Double cream	22	Bananas	130
Cheddar cheese	24	Milk	151
Sugar	25	Peas, boiled	204
Cornflakes	27	Apples	213
Pork sausages, fried	31	Oranges	286
Roast pork	32	Tomatoes	715
Beef steak, grilled	33		
Currants, dried	41		

The energy output of a man watching the television for two hours is approximately 180 Calories. If this man eats the following snacks during this two hours he takes in 712 Calories, ie he has taken in 532 Calories more than he has expended.

Snacks eaten

	Calories	kJ
1 cup of coffee		
1 tablespoonful of cream	30	126
2 teaspoonsful of sugar	40	168
1 can of beer	175	735
1 Mars bar	297	1247
Cheese biscuits	170	714
	712	2990

Energy

If 200 Calories are eaten every day for 1 year in excess of requirements of the body this results in a weight gain of the order of 10.88 kg (24 lb). 200 Calories can be represented by 4 cubes of chocolate, 50 g of sugar or 4 sweets. Walking 1 mile uses up 92 Calories and in order to lose 0.45 kg (1 lb) body fat 3000 Calories have to be expended. This can be done by walking 51.5 km (32 miles).

PRACTICAL WORK

1 Note how long you spend at various activities in 1 day. Using tables on energy expenditure which can be found in many physiology textbooks, work out how many Calories you expend in 1 day.
2 Weigh all food that you eat in a typical day, work out its Calorie content using food tables. Are you in positive or negative energy balance? ie are you taking in more Calories than you are expending or are you expending more Calories than you are taking in? Theoretically positive energy balance should result in an increase of body weight and negative energy balance should result in a loss of body weight.
3 Prepare 2 trays containing the following foods

Tray 1
50 g of fruit cake
10 g boiled sweets
10 g of sweet biscuits
85 g of sugar

Tray 2
100 g of lettuce
100 g of cucumber
100 g of tomatoes
100 g french or runner beans
100 g of grilled white fish
1 yogurt, plain
50 g of lean beef
1 apple or pear

Calculate from the food tables the Calorie value of each tray. What is the nutrient content of each tray? Which foods would be most suitable for a person on a reducing diet?

4 Make a list of foods which are high in their Calorific value but are important in the diet.
5 Make a list of foods which are high in Calories and can be safely omitted from the diet.
6 Make 100 Calorie (0.42 MJ) portions of some common foods to compare weights that supply 100 Calories.
7 Prepare a day's menu for an 18 year old girl who is trying to put on weight and secondly for an 18 year old girl who is trying to decrease her weight. Give weights of the foods to be eaten and calculate the Calorie values.
Prepare the meals and set out on trays.
8 Using a food calorimeter carry out experiments to determine the Calorie content of some common foods.

States of energy imbalance

1   If more energy is expended than is taken in there should be a loss in weight. This is the situation one is trying to achieve in a slimming diet.

2   Far more common is the situation in which more energy is taken in than is expended resulting in an increase in weight. Obesity affects a large proportion of the British population.

There are many ways of attacking the problem. Drugs can be used, exercise can be taken and surgical treatment can be given. The most sensible way to reduce weight is to eat a low carbohydrate diet. This involves cutting down on the sugary and starchy foods which are not essential for health. This diet can be used for years without harmful effects. A low protein diet cannot be used as proteins are vital in the body for repair of worn out cells and for growth in children. Fat intake can be reduced to some extent but some fat must be eaten to supply the essential fatty acids and the fat soluble vitamins.

A typical diet for 1 day for a young woman aged 23 years

Breakfast	Weight g	Calories	Kilojoules
Poached egg	50	81	340.2
Toast	35	105	441.0
Crispbread	7	30	126.0
Butter	15	119	499.8
Marmalade	10	26	109.2
Lunch			
Lettuce	10	1.1	4.62
Tomato	42	6	25.2
Cucumber	10	0.9	3.78
Cheese	80	340	1428
Fruit yoghurt	120	160	672
Jacket potato	100	84	352.8
Butter	10	79	331.8
Mid-afternoon			
Fruit cake	50	189	793.8
Supper			
½ grapefruit	100	11	46.2
Lamb chop	120	324	1360.8
Cauliflower	75	8	33.6
Carrots	75	15	63.0
Apple pie	75	142	596.4
Custard	50	58	243.6

Energy

Supper *continued*	Weight g	Calories	Kilojoules
Milk for day in coffee, tea, etc	400	264	1108.8
Sugar for day	10	38	159.6
Plain chocolate	30	181	760.2
		2262.0	9500.4

4
Protein, Fats and Carbohydrates

Proteins are the most important compounds present in living matter, without them life cannot exist. The word *protein* comes from a Greek word meaning 'to take first place'. Proteins are required by children for growth and repair and by adults for repair of the body's cells. All cells of the body need replacing at regular intervals as they only have a limited lifespan.

Protein malnutrition is the most widespread and serious nutritional deficiency disease in the world today.

The chemistry of proteins

All proteins contain the elements carbon, hydrogen, oxygen and nitrogen. Other elements such as phosphorus, sulphur and iron are often present. All proteins contain units called amino acids which are linked together by peptide bonds.

The simplest amino acid is glycine which has the following structure:

$$\mathrm{H - \underset{\underset{NH_2}{|}}{\overset{\overset{H}{|}}{C}} - COOH}$$

Amino acids are divided into two groups, the essential amino acids and the non-essential amino acids.

The essential amino acids

There are 8 essential amino acids; they are called essential because they must be supplied in the diet to keep the body healthy and they cannot be synthesised in the body. They are:

Methionine	Valine	Lysine	Phenylalanine
Tryptophan	Leucine	Threonine	Isoleucine

The best way to remember these names is to make up a sentence using the first one or two letters of each word.

There is one further amino acid called *histidine*, which is known to be essential for children.

Protein, Fats and Carbohydrates

The non-essential amino acids
There are twenty amino acids altogether; this number being made up with a group of amino acids which are called non-essential. These amino acids can be synthesised in the body provided the correct raw materials are present, and thus they do not have to be supplied in the diet. They are:

Alanine	Serine	Hydroxyproline	Aspartic acid
Arginine	Cystine	Tyrosine	Proline
Glycine	Cysteine	Glutamic Acid	

When protein foods are eaten they are broken down into amino acids in the process of digestion. The amino acids are absorbed in the small intestine and carried round in the blood circulation to the cells of the body where they are required for protein synthesis. The various cells of the body are able to manufacture specific types of protein, ie muscle cells will make muscle protein and the cells in the red bone marrow are able to manufacture protein for new red blood cells. Although there are only 20 different amino acids they are able to link together and form very complex molecules of protein. One amino acid can appear many times in one protein molecule. Every living organism makes protein that is distinctive for its species, eg the muscle protein of the dog is different from the muscle protein of humans. Protein makes up a high proportion of the solid matter of muscles, bones, teeth, hair, nails, skin, and the organs of the body such as the heart, lungs and liver.

Protein quality
A protein is said to be of good quality if it has an amino acid pattern similar to that of the tissues of the body. Proteins which contain the 8 essential amino acids in suitable proportions for tissue synthesis will be the most useful. The proteins which have the best quality protein are those from animal sources, the very best being egg protein and the protein in human milk.

Some proteins are lacking in one or more of the essential amino acids and these poor quality proteins cannot be used efficiently in the body. However, it is possible to eat two poor quality protein containing foods together and obtain a protein of good quality.

    eg   Protein food A is lacking in lysine but contains plenty of valine
            Protein food B is lacking in valine but contains plenty of lysine

If these two protein foods are eaten together at the same meal there is a supplementary effect and the deficiencies of the amino acids are counteracted and a good quality protein food is obtained.

Wheat has an insufficient quantity of lysine and thus lysine is called its limiting amino acid. When bread is eaten with cheese the lysine in cheese makes up for the lack of lysine in the flour.

Vegetable proteins tend to be of poor quality, but if two are eaten together there is usually a supplementary effect.

Food Sources of Protein

The staple food in most countries is one of the cereals — rice, wheat, maize or millet. These cereals contain reasonable amounts of protein of fair quality. But in some countries the staple foods are cassava, sweet potatoes, yams or plantains. All these foods are very low in their protein content and the protein that is present is of poor quality. Cassava, for example, contains less than 1% protein and is eaten in many tropical countries where there are very few other items in the diet. Protein malnutrition is common in countries which have starchy roots and tubers as their staple food. Legumes — especially the soya bean, peas and lentils are very useful in the diets of the people in poorer countries to supplement their protein content. Where meat, fish, cheese, milk and eggs are eaten in the diet there is no danger of protein deficiency.

In order to remember the protein content of some common foods we find that approximately 7 g of protein can be obtained from each of the following food portions:

187 ml (⅓ pint) of milk
28 g (1 oz) of beef steak (grilled)
28 g (1 oz) of cheese
28 g (1 oz) of grilled cod
1 egg

Food sources of protein

Good sources	% of protein	Poor sources	% of protein
Soya, full fat flour	40.3	Butter	0.4
Partridge, roast	35.2	Cream, double	1.5
Dried skimmed milk powder	34.5	Cooking oil	Trace
Chicken, roast	29.6	Apples	0.3
Peanuts	28.1	Oranges	0.8
Dried whole milk	27.0	Beans, runner, boiled	0.8
Cheese, cheddar	25.4	Marmalade	0.1
Beef steak, grilled	25.2	Sugar, white	Trace
Pork leg, roast	24.6	Lemonade	Trace
Cod, fried	20.7		
Sardines	20.4		
Cocoa powder	20.4		
Eggs	11.9		
Sausages, pork, fried	11.5		
Blended chocolate	9.2		
Peas, split dried, boiled	8.3		
Bread, white	8.3		
Milk	3.4		

Protein, Fats and Carbohydrates

Daily allowance of protein

Adult man   65 g – 90 g according to occupation
Adult woman   51 g – 63 g according to occupation
Pregnancy   60 g
Lactation   68 g

The daily allowance of protein for an adult woman can be obtained from

	g of protein
374 ml (⅔ pint) of milk	14
56 g (2 oz) cheese	14
112 g (4 oz) cod, grilled	28
50 g (approx 1 oz) of bread	4
	60

Thus there is no difficulty in obtaining enough protein in this country as we have a wide range of protein foods available.

A strict vegetarian (a vegan) who does not eat any foods of animal origin has considerable difficulty in obtaining enough protein. Vegetables do not contain such a high percentage of protein as the animal sources as they contain cellulose and more water. A vegan has to eat a wide range of vegetable foods in large portions in order to obtain enough protein.

A vegan could obtain 60 g of protein from the following foods

	g of protein
2 apples	0.6
2 bananas	2.2
100 g of peanuts	28.1
28g of soya flour	11.28
100 g bread, wholemeal	8.0
100 g peas, fresh boiled	5.0
50 g boiled lentils	3.4
100 g boiled potatoes	1.4
	59.98

Functions of proteins in the body
1   For growth.
2   To replace dead cells.
3   To synthesise the body's enzymes.
4   Protein can be used as a source of energy. If there is adequate fat and carbohydrate in the diet protein will be used for its primary functions, ie for growth and repair. If there are not enough energy containing foods in the diet, protein will be used to supply energy. In the diet of a carnivore a high proportion of the protein will be used to supply energy.

1 g of protein when completely oxidised in the body yields 4 Calories of energy (16.8 kJ).

Practical Work

Signs of deficiency of protein

When there is a lack of protein in the diets of children there will be a retardation of growth. If protein deficiency is prolonged the disease *Kwashiorkor* occurs. The name of this disease is from the Ga language of West Africa and means the disease by which the first child dies when the second child is born. In under-developed countries the infants are fed on human milk until they are 2 years old or even more. When the second child is born the first infant is often weaned on to a starchy gruel made from a food such as cassava which has a totally inadequate protein content. The first child can then suffer from kwashiorkor.

Symptoms of the disease are growth failure, loss of appetite, mental and physical apathy, a change in hair colour and texture, enlargement of the liver and muscle wasting. If the patient is put on to a protein rich diet recovery is rapid although irreparable damage may have been caused to the brain cells. Kwashiorkor mainly occurs in weaning infants and pre-school children.

PRACTICAL WORK

Make a list of the current retail prices for protein rich foods. Using the food tables calculate the cost of obtaining 100 g of protein from each food mentioned. Which food gives the best protein value for money? Does this food contain good quality protein?

Food	Cost per pound	Protein content g/oz	Cost per 100 g of protein
A	40p	5.0	$\frac{40}{16} \times \frac{100}{5.0} = 50\text{p}$

5.0 g of protein are present in 1 oz of food A

∴ 100 g of protein are present in $1 \times \frac{100}{5}$ oz of food A = 20 oz

16 oz of food A cost 40 p

∴ 20 oz of food A cost $40 \times \frac{20}{16}$ p = **50p**

or, expressed in metric calculations:

Food	Cost per kg	Protein content g/100 g	Cost per 100 g of protein
A	88p	17.6	$\frac{88}{1000} \times 100 \times \frac{100}{17.6}\text{p} = 50\text{p}$

17.6 g of protein are present in 100 g of food A

∴ 100 g of protein are present in $100 \times \frac{100}{17.6}$ g = 569 g of food A

1 kg (1000 g) of food A costs 88p

∴ 569 g of food A costs $88 \times \frac{569}{1000}$ p = **50 p**

Protein, Fats and Carbohydrates

Simulated meat protein

Simulated meat protein or textured vegetable protein is a food made from vegetable protein which has been modified to resemble meat. This meat has been on sale in the USA for some years and was originally designed for the vegetarian market.

Textured vegetable protein (TVP) is mainly made from soya bean flour as this contains a high percentage of good quality protein and provides a good yield per hectare. In this country TVP is made from field beans as these are grown here. 6 tonnes of field beans are needed to produce 1 tonne of protein which will be used to form 5 tonnes of TVP products. In the future it is expected that many acres of land in this country will be used for the cultivation of soya beans. There is a shortage of conventional meat supplies in many countries and TVP is becoming a feasible alternative. TVP is manufactured by two main methods:

1   Colour, flavour etc, are added to bean flour protein and the mixture is then heated with water and extruded under high pressure. The mixture is then expanded and dehydrated. The product has an open celled structure which on rehydration gives a product similar in colour, flavour and texture to that of meat.

2   This is a more expensive and complicated method. The bean flour protein is spun to form fibres. The fibres are coloured, flavoured, and assembled to simulate meat or chicken. If chicken is being made the muscle fibres will be assembled on a plastic carcass. The appearance of the product is good but the flavour and texture are usually criticised.

The TVP produced by the first method is at present about half the cost of conventional meat. The TVP produced by the second method is expensive but it is hoped that production costs will decrease.

TVP is finding a market in the UK in sausages, hamburgers, pies, curries, stews, ready-made meals and in pet foods. TVP presents no storage problems as it needs no refrigeration. When used in cooking it absorbs moisture and fat well and reduces cooking losses. It contains very little fat and no gristle. TVP is mainly used in conjunction with conventional meat to increase the protein content of dishes.

Nutritional value of a typical TVP sample compared with beef

	Hydrated TVP (30% solids)	Beef steak raw
Protein g	16.3	19.3
Water g	70.0	68.3
Fat g	0.3	10.5
Carbohydrate g	10.4	0.0
Calories	120	177

The nutritional value of TVP compares well with meat from conventional sources.

Textured Vegetable Protein tasting tests
Obtain samples of Textured Vegetable Protein from a health food stores. Prepare various dishes using TVP, eg curry, cottage pie, meat pie, sweet and sour pork, Bolognese sauce, etc. Also prepare the same dishes using conventional meat. Set up tasting panels to evaluate the taste, texture and flavour of TVP compared with conventional meat.

FATS IN THE DIET
Most of the fats eaten in the diet are triglycerides. But we also eat some phospholipids and steroids. All fats contain the elements carbon, hydrogen and oxygen.

Phospholipids
These are complex molecules often found in combination with protein. They play an important part in the structure of cell membranes and in fat metabolism. Lecithin, found in egg yolk, is a common phospholipid.

Steroids
The most important steroid is cholesterol which is synthesised in the body. Cholesterol is present in the blood and plays a necessary part in the transport of fatty acids. Cholesterol is found in all foods of animal origin. Eggs are exceptionally rich in their cholesterol content. Vegetables, fruit, nuts and cereals do not contain cholesterol.
The amount of cholesterol circulating in the bloodstream is affected by the diet. Egg yolks, animal fats and sucrose are amongst those foods which are known to increase blood cholesterol levels. A high blood cholesterol level is associated with thrombosis as this fatty substance together with other fats can become deposited inside the walls of arteries. Blood clots can develop on these fatty deposits and cause thrombosis by blocking off arteries. Coronary thrombosis occurs when a blood clot blocks off a coronary artery. Coronary thrombosis is a major killer and although there are many causative factors, faulty diet is one of them.
Many people with a history of thrombosis are having to eat a modified diet. They must cut down on their intake of animal fats, eggs and sugar, but they can consume vegetable oils which have a high proportion of unsaturated fatty acids which decrease blood cholesterol levels.

Triglycerides
Triglycerides account for about 98% of our dietary fat. They consist of 1 molecule of glycerol which has combined with 3 fatty acid molecules.

Protein, Fats and Carbohydrates

The formula for glycerol is:

```
      H
      |
H — C — OH
      |
H — C — OH
      |
H — C — OH
      |
      H
```

Glycerol, or glycerine is a very sweet substance, it is used in confectionary to increase creaminess and to prevent drying.

A simple triglyceride is formed when 3 molecules of the same fatty acid combine with glycerol.

```
     H                                    H
     |                                    |
H — C — OH      HOOC C3H7           H — C — O.CO.C3H7
     |                                    |
H — C — OH  +   HOOC C3H7   ⟶      H — C — O.CO.C3H7   + 3 H2O
     |                                    |
H — C — OH      HOOC C3H7           H — C — O.CO.C3H7
     |                                    |
     H                                    H
  Glycerol     3 molecules of            Tributyrin
               butyric acid
```

Most oils and fats contain different fatty acids and are called mixed triglycerides.

```
     H
     |
H — C — O.CO.A
     |                    A, B and C represent 3 different
H — C — O.CO.B            fatty acids
     |
H — C — O.CO.C
     |
     H
```

It is the fatty acids present in the triglyceride that determine the properties of the fat.

Saturated fatty acids

All fatty acids are composed of straight carbon chains. The saturated fatty acids are 'saturated' with hydrogen. Each carbon atom except for the two terminal ones combines with two hydrogen atoms.

Fats in the Diet

Butyric acid

```
      H   H   H
      |   |   |
  H — C — C — C — COOH        COOH is the acid grouping
      |   |   |
      H   H   H
```

Other examples of saturated fatty acids are caproic acid, lauric acid, myristic acid, palmitic acid and stearic acid.

Palmitic acid has the formula $C_{15}H_{31}COOH$ and is present in most fats. The saturated fatty acids predominate in triglycerides from animal sources. The hardness of a fat and its melting point increase as the proportion of saturated fatty acids increases. Suet, lard and meat fat contain mainly saturated fatty acids and thus they have a high melting point and they are hard at room temperatures. Most fats are made from mixtures of triglycerides, butter for example contains over twenty different fatty acids.

Unsaturated fatty acids

Some fatty acids have an insufficient number of hydrogen atoms to occupy all the carbon bonds. Where this occurs double bonds are found between carbon atoms. These fatty acids are said to be unsaturated, eg palmitoleic acid $CH_3 (CH_2)_5 CH = CH (CH_2)_7 COOH$.

```
    H   H   H   H   H   H   H   H   H   H   H   H   H   H   H
    |   |   |   |   |   |   |   |   |   |   |   |   |   |   |
H — C — C — C — C — C — C — C = C — C — C — C — C — C — C — C — COOH
    |   |   |   |   |               |   |   |   |   |   |   |
    H   H   H   H   H               H   H   H   H   H   H   H
```

Other unsaturated fatty acids are oleic acid $CH_3 (CH_2)_7 CH = CH (CH_2)_7 COOH$ which is the most common of all fatty acids, linoleic acid, arachidonic acid and linolenic acid. Fats with a high proportion of unsaturated fatty acids tend to be oils at room temperature. Vegetable oils contain predominantly unsaturated fatty acids. Unsaturated fatty acids are known to decrease blood cholesterol levels.

Essential fatty acids

There are 3 fatty acids which are known to be essential for normal functioning of the body. They are linoleic, linolenic and arachidonic acids.

Linoleic acid cannot be synthesised in the body and therefore must be supplied in the diet. Linolenic and arachidonic acids can be made from linoleic acid. A deficiency of essential fatty acids results in skin disorders. Linoleic acid is found in many vegetable oils, eg cottonseed, soya bean and sunflower seed oils.

Protein, Fats and Carbohydrates

Daily allowance of fat
   Most people in this country consume around 35% of their Caloric intake as fat. Thus a man on a diet of 3000 Cals will take in 1050 Cals as fat. Since 1 g of fat produces 9 Cals of energy in the body, this man will eat 117 g of fat. This figure is more than is necessary to meet the requirements of the body.

Functions of fat in the diet
1   Fat is primarily a source of energy, it provides 9 Calories of energy for each gramme of fat that is oxidised in the body. Fat is useful for reducing the bulk of the diet.
2   Fats contain the essential fatty acids which are essential for the health of the body.
3   Fats have a high satiety value due to the enterogastrone reflex. When fat is present in the stomach the hormone enterogastrone is released and this delays gastric emptying. Thus after a meal containing a high percentage of fat the onset of hunger is slow.
4   Fat improves the palatability of the diet. Many of our dishes would be tasteless if fat was omitted from them. Fat acts as a solvent for many of the food flavours.
5   Fat is a vehicle for the fat soluble vitamins A, D, E and K.
6   Fat forms a protective layer round the internal organs and acts as a heat insulator.

% Fat content of foods

Lard	99	Eggs	12.3
Suet	99	Ice cream	11.3
Margarine	85.3	Olives	11
Butter	85.1	Avocado pears	8
Almonds	53.5	Chicken, roast	7.3
Bacon, back, fried	53.4	Salmon, canned	6.0
Walnuts	51.5	Milk	3.7
Potato crisps	37.6	Apples	Trace
Milk chocolate	37.6	Oranges	Trace
Cheese, Cheddar	34.5	Sugar	0
Beef steak, grilled	21.6		
Mutton, leg roast	20.4		

CARBOHYDRATES IN THE DIET
   Carbohydrates include the starches, sugars, cellulose, pectins, dextrin, inulin and glycogen. All carbohydrates contain carbon, hydrogen and oxygen. There are two atoms of hydrogen for every one of carbon and oxygen. The simplest carbohydrates are the sugars and these are classified as monosaccharides or disaccharides. The sugars which are commonly found in the human diet are as follows:

Monosaccharides
1 *Glucose or dextrose* This has the chemical formula $C_6H_{12}O_6$ which has the structure:

Glucose is a white crystalline compound which is freely soluble in water. It is found in fruits and some vegetables. Glucose is the sugar which exists in the free state in the human blood and it serves as an indispensable source of energy for brain tissue in which little carbohydrate is stored.
2 *Fructose* is a white crystalline solid which has the chemical formula $C_6H_{12}O_6$.

Fructose is the sweetest of all sugars and is found in honey and ripe fruits.
3 *Galactose* is found as part of the disaccharide lactose, it does not exist on its own.

Disaccharides
1 *Maltose* consists of two glucose molecules linked together. It is found in cereals and beer.

It is the intermediate product in the digestion of starch into glucose.

STARCH $\xrightarrow{\text{amylase}}$ MALTOSE $\xrightarrow{\text{maltase}}$ GLUCOSE

2 *Lactose* This sugar consists of one glucose molecule and one galactose molecule linked together.

It is found in mammalian milk and is only mildly sweet.
3   *Sucrose* is the most important sugar in the diet. It is extracted from sugar cane and sugar beet. The chemical formula is $C_{12}H_{22}O_{11}$ and it consists of one molecule of glucose linked to one molecule of fructose.

The consumption of sucrose in this country has increased 25 times during the last two hundred years. The annual consumption per head is now about 50 kg or the weekly intake of sugar per head is about 0.91 kg (2 lb).

Sugar satisfies our palates rather than our dietary needs. It provides a cheap source of Calories but no other nutrients and can easily spoil the appetite for more valuable foods. Sucrose is consumed in a wide variety of foods — sweets, chocolates, biscuits, cakes, jellies, ice-cream, soft drinks, jams, canned fruit, etc, making it very difficult to avoid in the diet. There is evidence that sucrose contributes to dental caries, obesity, diabetes, and coronary thrombosis.

Sucrose provides 18% of our total Calorie intake per day.

Polysaccharides

These are the more complex carbohydrates which consist of many monosaccharide units linked together.
1   *Glycogen* is the reserve form of carbohydrate stored in the human body. 100 g of glycogen may be found in the liver and muscle. Glycogen is soluble in water and can be readily broken down into glucose in the body when there is a need for energy.
2   *Pectin* is the name given to a group of polysaccharides which are found in fruits and some vegetables. They are useful in that they form a gel in jam and jelly making.
3   *Dextrin* is a complex polysaccharide formed when starch is heated.
4   *Agar* is a polysaccharide extracted from seaweed and is used in food manufacture.
5   *Cellulose* is found in the cell wall of plants and gives support to the plant.

There are no enzymes in the human digestive tract which are able to digest cellulose so no energy is derived from it. Cellulose is useful in the diet as roughage.

6   *Starch* is the most valuable carbohydrate in the diet. It is eaten in large quantities in the staple food of many countries, ie as wheat, rice, maize, potatoes and cassava. Starch is found within the cellulose cell wall of plants and thus is not readily available in raw foods. On cooking the starch granules swell and rupture the cell walls, the cellulose is softened so the starch is available for digestion.

Average daily intake of carbohydrates

Starch	175 g
Sucrose	140 g
Lactose	20 g
Fructose	10 g
Glucose	5 g
	350 g → 1400 Calories

Carbohydrates provide about 50% of our Calories per day; in some countries they may provide 90% of the Calorie intake. Carbohydrates give a very high energy yield per hectare, they are easy to grow and palatable.

Most carbohydrates from natural sources carry with them a substantial quantity of vitamins, minerals and small quantities of protein. The potato is a useful food in this respect.

The intake of carbohydrates in the diet can be reduced without harmful effects to the health of the body and this is the most sensible way of reducing the Calorie intake in a slimming diet.

Function of carbohydrates in the diet
1   To provide energy. 1 g of carbohydrate when completely oxidised in the body provides approximately 4 Calories of energy.
2   They prevent the misuse of dietary protein for meeting energy requirements.

Excess carbohydrate in the diet is converted to the unflattering fat.

Chemical tests for proteins, fats and carbohydrates

PROTEINS
Million's Test
   To a sample of protein in a test tube add a few ml of Millon's Reagent. Boil the mixture, a reddish-pink precipitate indicates the presence of protein.
Biuret Test for protein molecules with 2 or more peptide bonds
   Place a few ml of protein solution in a test tube, add a few ml of 5% sodium hydroxide solution and a few ml of 1% copper sulphate solution. A pink or mauve colour is positive for molecules with 2 or more peptide bonds.

Protein, Fats and Carbohydrates

Percentage of energy derived from the protein, fat and carbohydrate in the diet of the average household – 1950-1971
(National Food Survey – Ministry of Agriculture, Fisheries and Food)

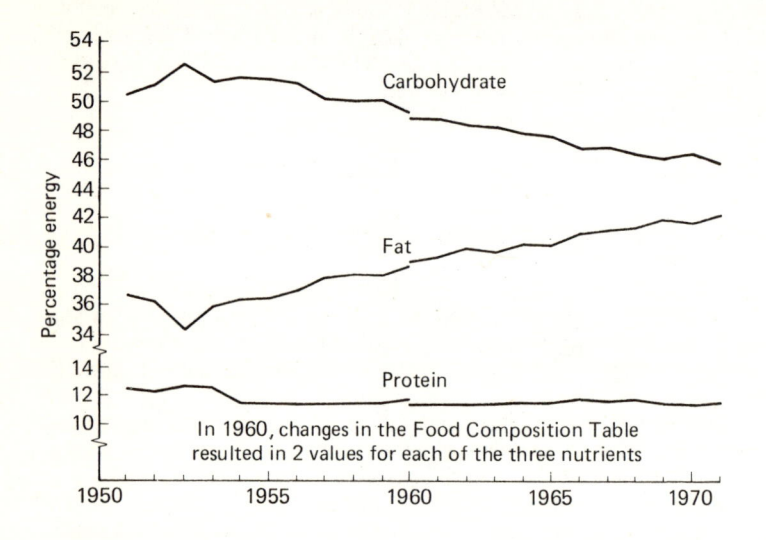

[Graph: Percentage energy (y-axis) vs year 1950–1970 (x-axis). Carbohydrate declines from ~50 to ~46; Fat rises from ~36 to ~42; Protein roughly constant ~12. Note: In 1960, changes in the Food Composition Table resulted in 2 values for each of the three nutrients]

FATS
Filter paper test
　　The presence of fat in a food sample can often be detected if when the sample comes into contact with filter paper it makes a translucent stain.
Osmium tetroxide test
　　Add a few drops of osmium tetroxide to the food sample, a black colour is formed if fat is present.
Sudan III test
　　Place a small quantity of starch in one test tube and an equal quantity of the food sample in a second test tube. Half fill each test tube with Sudan III solution, shake and filter. Observe the two residues left on the filter papers after they have dried. If the food sample contains fat the Sudan III will have stained it orange as compared with the pink colour of the fat free starch.

Chemical Tests for Carbohydrates

CARBOHYDRATES
Molisch's test
   Place a few ml of a carbohydrate solution in a test tube, add a few drops of alpha naphthol solution. Add a few drops of concentrated sulphuric acid solution very slowly. A purple ring formed at the junction of the liquids indicates the presence of a carbohydrate. This test is positive for all carbohydrates.

Iodine test
   Add a few drops of iodine solution to a sample of food containing starch. The formation of a blue-black colour is positive for starch.

Fehling's test
   To 3 ml of food sample add a few drops of Fehling's solutions A and B. Boil the mixture, a brick red precipitate will develop if sugars with reducing groups are present, eg glucose, fructose, lactose and maltose. The test is negative for sucrose.

Osazone test
   This test is used to distinguish between the different sugars.
   Half fill a test tube with a food sample solution, add a small spatula-full of phenylhydrazine hydrochloride and 2 small spatula-fuls of sodium acetate. Shake the mixture and heat until the solids have dissolved. Add 10 drops of glacial acetic acid and place the tube in a boiling water bath for 15 minutes. Cool and place a few crystals on a microscope slide and observe their shape under the microscope.
   Glucose and fructose form long slender crystals arranged in sheaves. These crystals usually develop in the water bath before cooling.
   Maltose forms flat crystals which can be arranged in rosettes.
   Lactose forms small thin crystals arranged like mimosa flowers.

5
Vitamins

The vitamins are vital substances required for the health of the body. They are needed in very small amounts, but since most foods only contain very small quantities of the vitamins care has to be taken to ensure that no vitamin deficiencies occur.

The vitamins are usually divided into 2 groups.
1   The fat soluble vitamins A, D, E and K.
2   The water soluble vitamins B and C.

VITAMIN A   RETINOL
This vitamin was originally found in milk. When rats were fed on a diet lacking in vitamin A they did not thrive but when milk was added to their diet they grew well. Vitamin A was isolated from milk as a pale yellow crystalline substance called retinol. A yellow substance called *carotene* was found to have the same effect as vitamin A in the body; this is because carotene is converted into vitamin A in the body.

Functions of vitamin A in the body
1   The maintenance of epithelial tissues lining the respiratory and urino-genital tracts. If there is a lack of vitamin A these lining cells become dry and scaly and an infection can easily set in.
2   To maintain the cells of the cornea of the eye.
3   To promote growth.

Signs of deficiency of vitamin A
1   Infection in certain epithelial cells.
2   Nightblindness. This is a failure of the eye to adapt to see in dim light.
   If a person suffering from nightblindness goes from bright sunlight into a darkened room they are unable to see anything even if they stay in the room for a length of time. If there is a prolonged lack of vitamin A in the diet the moist protective tissue of the eye becomes dry and thickened resulting in xerophthalmia. If vitamin A deficiency continues blindness can occur. Vitamin A deficiency is the cause of many cases of blindness in the under-developed countries.

Vitamin A

Daily allowance of vitamin A
750 µg for an adult
750 µg during pregnancy
1200 µg during lactation

The conversion of carotene to vitamin A in the body is not very efficient. It seems one needs to consume about 6 µg of carotene to make 1 µg of vitamin A in the body. Vitamin A can be stored in the body in the liver, so it is not necessary to have vitamin A every day in the diet.

Food sources of vitamin A
In Great Britain one third of our vitamin A comes from animal sources in the form of vitamin A and two thirds comes as carotene from vegetable sources.

per 100 g of food	µg of vit A
Cod liver oil	22740
Fried liver, ox	6600
Butter	1050
Cheese	420
Kidney	300
Eggs	300
Herring	45
Milk	30-45
Plain yoghurt	14
Dried skimmed milk	Trace

There is virtually no vitamin A in beef, chicken, pork, lamb or white fish.

Sources of carotene measured in µg per 100 g of food

Carrots	6000-12000
Watercress	3000
Apricots	1500
Lettuce	1000
Prunes	500
Oranges	50

Effect of cooking on vitamin A
Vitamin A is quite stable even when food is boiled for a long time. During frying when the temperature is high and oxygen is present some vitamin A is destroyed.

Hypervitaminosis A
As vitamin A can be stored in the liver it is possible to suffer from an overdose. This could occur if an excess of halibut liver oil or cod liver oil is consumed. The symptoms are varied, the bones may become

Vitamins

soft, there is an increased tendency to bleed, the skin becomes dry and the hair coarse and sparse.

VITAMIN D (chemical name *cholecalciferol*)
Vitamin D was first used as a remedy for the disease rickets in the form of cod liver oil in the eighteenth century. Vitamin D is obtained by the body in two ways, firstly by ingestion of certain foods and secondly it is formed under the skin from its precursor 7-dehydrocholesterol when the skin is exposed to sunlight.

Functions of vitamin D in the body
Vitamin D is concerned with the absorption of calcium and phosphorus from the intestine and their deposition in the bones and teeth.

Signs of deficiency of vitamin D
1 The main sign of a lack of this vitamin is the bone disease rickets. This disease has been known for 2-3000 years and used to be very common in this country. Rickets was common because diets were low in vitamin D and calcium, children were not often exposed to the sunlight and the atmosphere was so polluted that the sun's rays that reached the earth were not powerful. The incidence of rickets is now low in this country.
The disease rickets is characterised by a thickening of the joints, pigeon chest, bossing of the skull and bow legs or knock knees. The adult form of rickets is called osteomalacia and occurs due to the lack of vitamin D and calcium in the diet, lack of sunshine and repeated pregnancies in women.
2 Dental caries. If there is inadequate calcium absorption then the teeth will be poorly calcified resulting in dental caries.

Daily allowance of vitamin D
This cannot be accurately established as it is not known how much vitamin D is synthesised under the skin.
The recommended dietary intake for adults is 2.5 μg and 10 μg during pregnancy and lactation.

Food sources of vitamin D

per 100 g	μg of vit D
Cod liver oil	218
Herring	22.5
Sardines	7.5
Margarine	7.5
Eggs	4.25
Ox liver	1.1
Butter	1.0
Cheese	0.3

There is no vitamin D in pork, beef, lamb, chicken, white fish, fruit, vegetables, nuts and cereals.

Effect of cooking on vitamin D
Vitamin D is stable to light and heat and is well retained in most methods of food preparation.

Hypervitaminosis D
Vitamin D like vitamin A, is stored in the body and excessive amounts can build up. Signs of hypervitaminosis are nausea, anorexia and renal damage due to the deposition of calcium compounds in the kidneys.

VITAMIN E   (chemical name *Tocopherol*)
Vitamin E was discovered in 1923 in California when rats fed on a diet of casein, corn starch, yeast, butter and lard suffered from reproductive abnormalities. The male rats became sterile and the females aborted, when wheat germ oil was added to their diet the rats became fertile. The wheat germ oil was found to contain vitamin E.

Functions of vitamin E in the body
1   In many animals vitamin E is necessary for normal reproduction. There is no conclusive evidence that it is required for normal reproduction in humans.
2   It is concerned with oxidation reactions in the cell.

Signs of deficiency of vitamin E
There are no easily recognisable signs of vitamin E deficiency in man.

Daily allowance of vitamin E
Since the functions of vitamin E are not clearly understood no recommended allowance can be given.

Food sources of vitamin E
Vitamin E is found in virtually every food, the richest sources are wheat germ oil, barley, rye, green vegetables, oatmeal, eggs, meat, margarine, liver and butter.

mg of vitamin E per 100 g of food	
Peas, raw	2.1
Eggs	2.0
Bread, wholemeal	1.9
Butter	1.9
Liver, ox	1.4
Mutton and lamb	0.8
Apples	0.7
Tomatoes	0.4

Vitamins

VITAMIN K (chemical name *naphthoquinone*)
In 1934 vitamin K was found to prevent a haemorrhagic disease of chickens.

Function of vitamin K in the body
Vitamin K is necessary for normal blood clotting. It is used to aid the manufacture of prothrombin in the liver.

Signs of vitamin K deficiency
An abnormal clotting time of the blood. A lack of vitamin K in adults is extremely unusual as even poor diets seem to contain an adequate amount of vitamin K. Vitamin K is produced by the intestinal flora and this source may provide enough for bodily needs. In the new-born baby there can be haemorrhagic disorders which are due to a lack of vitamin K.

Daily allowance of vitamin K
There are no recommended intakes for this vitamin as it is very unlikely that a deficiency will occur. An unmeasurable amount of vitamin K is synthesised in the intestine.

Food sources of vitamin K
Dark green vegetables, tomatoes, egg yolk and liver are the best sources.

mg of vitamin K per 100 g of food	
Spinach	4.2
Green cabbage	3.2
Tomatoes	0.4
Ox liver	0.1-0.2
Lean meat	0.1-0.2
Eggs	0.04

WATER SOLUBLE VITAMINS

THE B COMPLEX
Here we shall deal only with the well known vitamins of this group.

Vitamin B1   Thiamine
This vitamin was discovered in 1887 when Takaki, Director of Japanese sailors, had a large number of sailors suffering from the disease known as beri-beri. These sailors were given wheat and milk in their diet and they recovered. Their recovery was later shown to be due to the presence of vitamin B1 mainly in the wheat.
In 1891 Eijkman showed that unpolished rice could restore his

Vitamin B1

beri-beri patients to good health. Later it was found that there was a substance in the husk of rice which prevented beri-beri and that most of this substance was removed when rice was milled. This substance was called thiamine or vitamin B1. It is a white crystalline compound which is highly soluble in water.

Functions of B1 in the body
1 It is used in reactions leading to the release of energy from carbohydrates.
2 It promotes nerve activity.

Signs of deficiency of B1
Firstly there may be a loss of appetite, irritability and tiredness. If the deficiency of B1 is prolonged the disease beri-beri will develop which primarily affects the nervous system. This disease is common in rice eating communities where the diet is poor and made up of a large percentage of milled rice.

There are three forms of beri-beri. 1 Wet beri-beri. 2 Dry beri-beri. 3 Infant beri-beri.
1 *Wet beri-beri* The patient suffers from oedema, palpitations and pain in the limbs. Carbohydrates are incompletely metabolised and lactic acid and pyruvic acid accumulate, these dilate the blood vessels, fluid leaks through the capillaries and oedema occurs. Death can occur through heart strain.
2 *Dry beri-beri* In this form of the disease there is no oedema but there is severe wasting of the muscles and often paralysis. Dry beri-beri can develop into the more serious wet beri-beri.
3 *Infant beri-beri* This occurs in babies aged 1-6 months due to the mother's milk being deficient in B1; this will happen if the mother's diet is poor in its B1 content. The infant may die of heart failure. Recovery is amazingly rapid once B1 is administered.

The incidence of beri-beri can be decreased if rice is not dehusked and polished but unfortunately unpolished rice is not popular.

Daily allowance of B1
For adults 1.0 mg per day.
If the diet is high in its carbohydrate content then there is a greater need for thiamine to ensure that the carbohydrate is completely metabolised.

Food sources of B1
B1 is found in nearly all animal and plant tissues.

Vitamins

	mg of B1 per 100 g of food
Yeast, bakers, dried	6-24
Peanuts	0.9
Pork, roast	0.8
Bacon	0.4
Liver	0.3
Peas, boiled	0.25
Bread, wholemeal	0.20
Bread, white	0.18
Salmon, raw	0.10
Eggs	0.10
Sultanas	0.10
Oranges	0.10
Potatoes, boiled	0.08
White fish, raw	0.06
Milk	0.04
Cheese, cheddar	0.04

Milled cereals are low in their thiamine content. In this country thiamine is added to all white flour to ensure that the population gets a reasonable intake of thiamine from its staple food.

Effect of cooking on B1
Vitamin B1 is destroyed by high temperatures and is very soluble in water so considerable losses can take place in food preparation. Its destruction is speeded up in an alkaline environment, eg in some baked products.

VITAMIN B2   RIBOFLAVIN
This yellow crystalline compound was isolated from milk in 1933, but has since been found in liver, eggs, green leafy and yellow vegetables.

Functions of B2 in the body
B2 is essential for cell respiration. It is also necessary for the maintenance of mucosal and eye tissues.

Signs of deficiency of B2
There is no definite deficiency disease associated with a lack of B2. The term ariboflavinosis is used to describe the symptoms which occur. Shortage of B2 leads to a failure of the appetite, stunted growth, cracks and sores and burning sensations about the nose and mouth and a sensation of grittiness under the eyelids. Ariboflavinosis occurs in many parts of the world where the diet is poor but it is not a fatal disease.

Daily allowance of B2
1.5 mg for an adult.

Food sources of B2

	mg of B2 per 100 g of food
Liver, raw	3.0
Yeast, bakers, dried	17.8
Cheese, cheddar	0.5
Chocolate	0.35
Eggs	0.35
Mushrooms, fried	0.35
Milk	0.15
Spinach, boiled	0.15
Peas, boiled	0.11
Bread, wholemeal	0.10
Peanuts	0.10
Bananas	0.07
Apricots, dried, stewed	0.06

Effect of cooking on B2

B2 is more stable to heat than B1 but it tends to be destroyed by sunlight. Exposure of milk to sunlight for 2 hours results in a 50% loss of B2.

VITAMIN B3   PANTOTHENIC ACID

Pantothenic acid is found in virtually all foods and thus no clear definition of its deficiency signs in humans are available. It is essential in cell metabolism.

NICOTINIC ACID

Nicotinic acid was isolated from yeast in 1913 and subsequently nicotinic acid was found to be effective in the treatment of the disease called pellagra in humans and black tongue in dogs.

Functions of nicotinic acid in the body

It is essential for cell metabolism.

Signs of deficiency of nicotinic acid

The disease pellagra is caused through lack of nicotinic acid. This disease was first described in 1730 amongst peasants in Spain who had maize as their staple food. This disease occurs in North Africa, Yugoslavia, South America and Southern Italy where maize is the staple food.

The word *pellagra* is Italian, meaning 'sour skin'. The clinical signs of pellagra are the 'three Ds' dermatitis, diarrhoea and dementia. The dermatitis occurs mostly on skin surfaces exposed to the sun. The intestinal tract becomes inflamed and diarrhoea occurs and there are psychic changes causing hallucinations and depression.

Vitamins

When maize is analysed for its nicotinic acid content it is found to have enough nicotinic acid to prevent pellagra. This remained a problem for some time until it was found that the nicotinic acid in maize was in a bound form called niacytin and this compound is not absorbed in the intestinal tract; thus the maize eaters were suffering from pellagra.

Maize eaters in Mexico do not suffer from pellagra as they soak the maize in lime water to help remove the husk and this soaking in an alkali releases the nicotinic acid from the niacytin.

Some foods which are rich in tryptophan have an anti-pellagra effect. This is because tryptophan can be converted into nicotinic acid in the body.

Daily allowance of nicotinic acid
For adults 18 mg per day.

Food sources of nicotinic acid

mg of nicotinic acid per 100 g of food

Liver, fried	15
Chicken, roast	6
Beef, roast	5
Mushrooms, fried	3.5
Wholemeal bread	3.5
Cod	3.0
White bread	1.7
Bacon, fried	1.5
Potatoes, boiled	0.8

Effect of cooking on nicotinic acid
Nicotinic acid is resistant to moderate heat, light, oxidation and alkalis. Thus it survives cooking quite well although some can be lost in the cooking water.

VITAMIN B6   PYRIDOXINE
This vitamin was isolated in 1938 as a factor which would cure a skin disease in rats.

Functions of B6 in the body
B6 is essential for protein, fat and carbohydrate metabolism and for the metabolism of nervous tissue.

Signs of deficiency of B6
Deficiency of B6 is very rare. Some cases have been found in infants when they have been fed with overheated milk in which the B6 has largely been destroyed. The main sign of deficiency is convulsions.

Vitamin B6

Daily allowance of B6
Most diets provide 1-2 mg per day and since there are no signs of deficiency in Great Britain it is thought that this amount is adequate.

Food sources of B6
Yeast, liver, herring, rice polishings, germ of grains, seeds and egg yolks.

Effect of cooking on B6
Some B6 is lost by the heat of cooking.

FOLIC ACID
This substance is found in leafy vegetables, liver, kidneys and yeast. It is important in nutrition as it is an essential part of red blood cells and is used in protein metabolism. A deficiency gives rise to a megaloblastic anaemia, a disorder in which the red blood cell count is decreased and the red blood cells are mis-shapen and fragile.

VITAMIN B12   CYANOCOBALAMIN
This vitamin is a red crystalline substance containing cobalt. It had been known for some years that patients suffering from pernicious anaemia could be helped if they ate raw liver; but it was not until 1948 that B12 was isolated and found to be the active factor in liver. To obtain 1 g of B12 50 tonnes of liver were required. The complex chemical structure of B12 was determined in 1955.

Functions of B12 in the body
B12 plays a vital part in certain enzyme systems. It is necessary for the formation of normal red blood cells.

Signs of deficiency of B12
B12 deficiency is usually due to a failure to absorb the vitamin rather than a dietary deficiency. A protein substance called the intrinsic factor has to be present in the stomach before B12 can be absorbed. In the B12 deficiency disease, pernicious anaemia, the stomach does not produce the intrinsic factor and B12 is not absorbed from the food. The result is that the red blood cells are abnormal, pernicious anaemia is a type of megaloblastic anaemia. Control of this disease is by injections of B12.

Daily allowance of B12
3-4 μg per day for an adult.

Vitamins

Food sources of B12

	µg per 100 g of food
Liver, ox	50
Herring	10
Mutton and lamb	2.0
Pork	2.0
Beef	2.0
Cod	1.0
Eggs	0.7
Milk	0.3

Vitamin B12 is not found in plant foods and thus strict vegetarians do not get a dietary source of B12.

Effect of cooking on B12
Some B12 is lost by the heat of cooking.

VITAMIN C   ASCORBIC ACID
Vitamin C is a white crystalline carbohydrate which is very soluble in water. The deficiency disease associated with vitamin C is scurvy and this used to be very common amongst sailors and men on expeditions. James Lind, a naval surgeon in 1757 noted that scurvy could be controlled amongst his sailors if they were given citrus fruits in addition to their normal diets. The factor in citrus fruits which was anti-scorbutic was isolated as Ascorbic acid in about 1932.

Functions of vitamin C in the body
1   Vitamin C is connected with the synthesis of collagen, which is the substance which acts as a cement between the cells of the body and also holds the bones and teeth together.
2   Vitamin C acts in many enzyme reactions and is closely involved in the metabolism of proteins, carbohydrates and fats.
3   It aids the absorption of iron from the diet.
4   The connection between vitamin C intake and the common cold has not been clearly elucidated.

Signs of deficiency of vitamin C
In the first stages of scurvy there is general tiredness and weakness and then pinprick haemorrhages appear under the skin. Later as the deficiency proceeds the gums redden and swell, any wounds heal very slowly, teeth may weaken and fall out and anaemia often occurs. In this disease old wounds can open up and previous bone breaks can recur.

The disease scurvy is uncommon in underdeveloped countries where there is usually a good supply of fresh fruits and vegetables. A surprisingly large number of old people are suffering from mild forms of scurvy in Great Britain.

Vitamin C

Daily allowance of vitamin C

There is a great deal of controversy about the requirements for vitamin C. In this country the daily allowance recommended for adults is 30 mg. More vitamin C should be given after surgery to aid the healing process and the absorption of iron.

Food sources of vitamin C

Vitamin C is primarily found in fruit and vegetables. There is a very small amount in fresh meat and milk. Rosehip syrup and blackcurrant juice or puree are very useful in the diets of people who are likely to be lacking in vitamin C. Potatoes are an important source of vitamin C because of the quantity consumed. Fresh potatoes contain 30 mg of vitamin C per 100 g but this value falls on storage.

mg of vit C per 100 g of food		mg of vit C per 100 g of food	
Blackcurrants, raw	200	Liver, fried	20
Rosehip syrup	150	Blackberries, raw	20
Parsley	150	Cabbage, boiled	20
Horseradish	120	Tomatoes, raw	20
Mustard and cress	80	Lettuce	15
Strawberries	60	Peas, boiled	15
Cabbage, raw	60	Potatoes, new, boiled	15-21
Watercress	60	Potatoes, old, boiled	4.0-5.6
Oranges	50	Parsnips, boiled	10
Lemons	50	Bananas	10
Grapefruit	40	Peaches, raw	8
Melon	25	Apples	5
Pineapple	25	Pears, raw	3
Raspberries	25	Milk	1.5

Effect of cooking and processing on vitamin C

Unfortunately vitamin C can easily be lost in cooking and processing as it is very soluble in cooking water and heat labile. For these reasons vitamin C rich foods must be cooked quickly in a minimum amount of water and where possible the cooking water should be used to make the gravy. Foods should not be cut up too much before they are cooked as cutting across the cell walls releases the vitamin C; and fruits and vegetables must not be soaked in water before they are cooked as the vitamin C will dissolve into the water. Fruits and vegetables must be eaten as soon as they are cooked, if they are kept warm before they are eaten the vitamin C content will be very small.

Vitamin C is well preserved in an acid environment. A small amount of vitamin C is lost when fruits and vegetables are blanched before they are frozen and some vitamin C is lost in the canning process.

Vitamins

PRACTICAL WORK

1   Prepare trays of foods showing how the daily allowance of vitamins A, D, B1 and C can be obtained.
2   Calculate your intake of the four vitamins given above in the food you ate yesterday.
3   Obtain a range of common vitamin C rich foods. Write down their vitamin C content per 100 g of the food using the food tables and weigh out suitable portions of each to give the daily allowance of vitamin C, ie 30 mg.
4   Calculate the cost of obtaining 30 mg of vitamin C from the fruits and vegetables provided. Show a comparison of the costs on a bar graph.
5   Take 1 kg (2.2 lb) of new potatoes and 1 kg (2.2 lb) of old potatoes. Prepare all potatoes for boiling. Weigh each sample of prepared potatoes. Calculate the percentage loss of weight which has occurred on preparing the potatoes.

Using the food tables calculate the vitamin C content of the edible portion of the prepared potatoes.

Carry out vitamin C estimations on a 5 g sample of the old and the new potatoes before and after boiling. Boil each sample in the same volume of water for the same length of time.

Taking current costs of potatoes into account and allowing for peeling losses is it more economical to obtain vitamin C from old or new potatoes?

Vitamin Intake

Name of Vitamin	Uses in the body	Deficiency signs	Sources	Daily recommended allowances for adults
A Retinol	Maintenance of epithelial tissues Growth	Nightblindness Xerophthalmia	Liver, butter, margarine, egg yolk, milk, oily fish As carotene – carrots, apricots, green vegetables	750 µg
D Cholecalciferol	Absorption of calcium and phosphorus Calcification of bones	Rickets Dental caries Osteomalcia	Sunlight Liver, egg yolk, milk, butter, margarine, oily fish	2.5 µg
E Tocopherol	Cell metabolism	Infertility in animals	Wheat germ oil, liver, egg yolk, milk, peanuts, vegetables	
K Naphthoquinone	Blood clotting	Haemorrhage	Spinach, cabbage, tomatoes, egg yolk, meat Intestinal flora	
B1 Thiamine	Carbohydrate metabolism	Beri-beri Skin hyperaesthesia	Yeast, wheat germ, liver, meat, peas, beans	1.0 mg
B2 Riboflavin	Energy release	Soreness and burning of lips, mouth and tongue Digestive disturbances	Yeast, marmite, liver, milk, beef, cheese	1.5 mg
Nicotinic acid	Energy release	Pellagra 3 Ds	Meat, fish, cereals	18 mg
B6 Pyridoxine	Metabolism	Convulsions	Yeast, liver, meat, cereals, fish	
B12 Cyanocobalamin	Red blood cell formation	Pernicious anaemia	Liver, herring, meat, fish, cheese, eggs, milk	3-4 µg
C Ascorbic acid	Maintenance of connective tissue	Scurvy	Blackcurrants, strawberries, rosehips, citrus fruit, parsley, green peppers, cabbage	30 mg

6
Minerals and Water

As we have seen, the body requires certain nutrients such as protein, fat and vitamins in order to stay healthy. Minerals are also necessary for health. They are widely distributed in nature and make up about 7% of the body-weight. The minerals are not found in their free state in foods, they are eaten as compounds, eg calcium may be eaten as calcium carbonate and sodium as sodium chloride. Minerals are found in the soil and rocks. Plants absorb them through their roots, animals eat the plants and obtain their mineral supply. Man can obtain his minerals from animal and plant foods. It must be noted that two samples of the same food can vary widely in their mineral content due to variations in the mineral content of the soil.

As the majority of the population eats a wide range of foods mineral deficiencies are not common, with the exception of iron deficiency anaemia. Some minerals are found in quite large quantities in the body, eg calcium and phosphorus compounds which are mainly found in the bones and teeth. Minerals which are present in very small quantities in the body are called trace elements. Examples of trace elements are iodine, fluorine, cobalt and copper.

Weight of some important minerals found in the body

Calcium	1200 g
Phosphorus	700 g
Potassium	245 g
Sulphur	170 g
Chlorine	120 g
Sodium	105 g
Magnesium	30 g
Iron	4 g

CALCIUM

Calcium is the most important inorganic element in the body and occurs in the largest amount. The body contains 1200 g of calcium, 99% of this is found in the bones and teeth and 1% in the soft tissues.

Calcium

Functions of calcium in the body
1   For the formation of bones and teeth. Bones consist of 60% calcium phosphate and 40% collagen and other soft tissues. Vitamin D must be present in the diet to aid the absorption of calcium from the small intestine and the deposition of calcium in the bones and teeth.
2   Calcium must be present in the blood to enable normal clotting to take place.
3   Calcium aids the clotting of milk in the stomach.
4   Calcium is necessary for the contraction of muscles.

Signs of deficiency of calcium
1   Teeth become decalcified.
2   Bones become decalcified and the disease rickets develops in children and osteomalacia in adults.

Recommended allowances
500 mg per day for adults
1200 mg per day during pregnancy and lactation
   The extra requirement for calcium during pregnancy is for the formation of bones and teeth in the foetus. During lactation there is a loss of 150-300 mg of calcium per day from the mother's body in the milk so there is an obvious need for more calcium in the diet. If the mother's intake of calcium is insufficient, calcium from her bones and teeth will be used for the foetus or for the milk, resulting in a weakening of their structure.

Absorption of calcium
   Unfortunately only 20-50% of the calcium eaten in the diet is actually absorbed, the rest is excreted in the faeces. It is essential that vitamin D is present to aid the absorption of calcium. There are certain substances present in food which make it difficult for the body to absorb calcium. Two such substances are phytic and oxalic acids. Phytic acid is present in the outer layers of cereal grains, it combines with calcium rendering it difficult for absorption to take place. The importance of this in the diet is a matter of great controversy. Oxalic acid found in rhubarb and spinach combines with calcium forming calcium oxalate which is also difficult to absorb.

Excretion of calcium
   Calcium is excreted mainly in the faeces but some is also lost in the urine and sweat.

Food sources of calcium
   The easiest way to obtain enough calcium is to drink ½ litre of milk per day as this provides 613 mg of calcium.

Minerals and Water

Calcium rich foods

Per 100 g	mg
Dried, skimmed milk	1265
Dried, whole milk	960
Cheddar cheese	810
Spinach, boiled	595
Sardines, canned	409
Parsley	325
Almonds	247
Soya flour	208
Broccoli	160
Milk	120
Bread, white	91
Haricot beans, boiled	64.5
Cabbage, winter, boiled	58
Eggs	56

Sardines and other canned fish are good sources of calcium as their soft bones are eaten.

The daily allowance of calcium could be obtained thus:

	mg of calcium
284 ml of milk	350
3 slices of white bread	78
50 g of boiled cabbage	29
100 g of fried plaice	44.9
100 g of stewed beef	3
	504.9

or thus

3 slices of white bread	78
75 g of chips	10.4
50 g of sardines	204
1 fruit yoghurt	227
	519.4

Bread is quite a good source of calcium as white flour is enriched with calcium carbonate by law.

If milk and cheese are liked there is no problem in getting enough calcium in the diet; but in the case of the vegan calcium must be obtained from nuts, cereals and green vegetables.

Effect of cooking on calcium

Mineral salts are not destroyed by cooking, but some calcium will be found in the cooking water especially in that of green vegetables. If this water is used for making gravy only a very small proportion of calcium will be lost. In hard water areas the calcium present in the water will increase the dietary intake of the mineral.

PHOSPHORUS
There are about 682 g (1½lb) of phosphorus in the body. 78% of it is found in the bones and teeth and 22% is found in the body fluids and soft tissues. Phosphorus is a very important element as it is present in every cell of the body and has numerous bodily functions.

Functions of phosphorus in the body
1 It is used in the formation of bones and teeth.
2 It plays a vital part in the metabolism of proteins, fats, carbohydrates and vitamins.
3 It is used in buffering systems to help regulate the pH of the blood.

Signs of deficiency of phosphorus
A deficiency of this mineral is extremely unlikely as all diets seem to contain enough. If there is enough calcium in the diet there will be adequate phosphorus. No specific deficiency disease has been noted in man.

Daily allowance of phosphorus
There are no figures given for phosphorus.

Food sources of phosphorus
These are numerous and similar to those containing calcium.

Phosphorus content per 100 g

	mg
Sardines	683
Cheddar cheese	545
Almonds	442
Eggs	218
Milk, fresh whole	95
Spinach, boiled	93
White bread	81

SODIUM
The body contains 105 g of sodium in the form of sodium chloride (salt), sodium bicarbonate and sodium phosphate. Sodium is mainly found in the body fluids. Salt is the only mineral compound for which the body has an appetite. Many people add large quantities of salt to their food to improve its flavour.

Functions of sodium in the body
1 Sodium helps to regulate the volume of the extra-cellular body fluids.
2 It helps to maintain acid-base balance in the body.
3 It is necessary for nerve conduction.

Minerals and Water

Signs of deficiency

Sodium deficiency can occur with dehydration as a result of heat exhaustion. The symptoms are muscular cramp, anorexia, lethargy and sickness. Sodium deficiency can occur amongst miners who work at high temperatures and lose a lot of water and salt through sweating. Thus sodium deficiency is commonly called *Miner's Cramp*. Cramp due to a lack of salt can also occur in athletes who are not used to performing at high temperatures. The remedy for Miner's cramp is to drink some water containing salt or to take salt tablets.

Sodium excess can result in oedema but this should not normally occur as excess salt is excreted.

Daily allowance of sodium

Only about 0.5 g of sodium is needed by the body each day. Most people consume 10-20 g per day.

Sodium is absorbed easily and rapidly. Excess sodium is excreted in the urine, sweat and faeces. The amount of sodium that is retained in the body is under the hormonal control of the adrenal gland.

Food sources of sodium

per 100 g	g
Bovril	4.55
Bacon, collar, fried	3.05
Ham, lean only	2.10
Haddock, smoked	1.22
Sausages, pork, fried	0.99
Cheese, cheddar	0.61
Bread, white	0.52
Eggs	0.14
Milk	0.05

Sodium is also eaten in the diet in the form of monosodium glutamate which is a common additive in soups, canned meat and Chinese food.

POTASSIUM

The human body contains 245 g of potassium and this is mostly found in the skeletal muscle. It is a predominant metal in the body's cells.

Functions of potassium in the body

1   Conduction of nervous impulses.
2   The maintenance of acid-base balance.
3   The maintenance of osmotic pressure in the body.

Signs of deficiency of potassium

Muscular weakness and paralysis. Deficiency can occur as a result of the protein deficiency disease, kwashiorkor. As the cells of the body are broken down in this disease during muscle wasting the body loses nitrogen and since the cells contain potassium this also is lost. Deficiency could also occur in starvation.

Daily allowance of potassium
Usually 2-5 g are taken in per day in a normal mixed diet and this seems adequate.

Potassium is excreted in the urine, faeces and sweat.

Food sources of potassium
All foods contain potassium. Dried fruits, nuts, meat, fish, cereals, chocolate and vegetables are good sources. Sugar, butter and margarine are poor sources.

MAGNESIUM
In 1618 water was found in Epsom which contained large amounts of magnesium sulphate (Epsom salts). This water was used as a purgative.

The body contains 20-30 g of magnesium mainly found in the bones as magnesium phosphate or bicarbonate. Magnesium is present in important amounts in the soft tissues of the body and is found in all cells.

Functions of magnesium in the body
1 It controls the irritability of muscles and nerves.
2 It is used in enzyme systems in metabolism.

Signs of deficiency of magnesium
Muscle tremor, tetany, convulsions and coma. Deficiency can occur in alcoholics and those with malabsorption disorders. Deficiency on a normal diet is very rare as all foods contain some magnesium.

Daily allowance of magnesium
300-400 mg seems to be adequate.

Food sources of magnesium
Magnesium is found in all foods. It is necessary in photosynthesis for the formation of chlorophyll and this will be in all green parts of the plant. Vegetarians will therefore have a high intake of magnesium. Cereals, green vegetables, nuts, soya beans and chocolate are good sources of magnesium.

IRON
Iron is of great importance in nutrition. It has been used therapeutically for many centuries. It was originally used for healing wounds but since the seventeenth century it has been used for curing and preventing iron deficiency anaemia. In the seventeenth century a large

Minerals and Water

number of adolescent girls suffered from an illness they called green sickness or love sickness. This illness was really anaemia. The girls were cured with a mixture of red wine, iron filings and sugar. Later on it was discovered that these disorders were a result of iron deficiency in the diet, but it was not known until 1932 that iron was a vital part of haemoglobin in the red blood corpuscles.

The adult body contains 4 g of iron. 2.5 g is present in the haemoglobin, some is in myoglobin in muscles and some is in the iron store in the form of the compounds haemosiderin and ferritin.

Functions of iron in the body
1   Iron is an essential part of the blood pigment haemoglobin which is in the red blood cells. Haemoglobin carries oxygen from the lungs to the cells of the body. The red corpuscles are made in the red bone marrow. A red blood cell has a life of 120 days and since there are about 5 million red blood cells in every cubic millimetre of blood it has been calculated that 200 000 million new cells have to be made every day. Hence there is a constant demand for iron.
2   Iron is used in the formation of the muscle pigment myoglobin, which can take up and release oxygen as it is required.
3   Iron is concerned with the transfer of oxygen in the cells.

Signs of deficiency of iron
The iron deficiency disease is iron deficiency anaemia. The symptoms are tiredness, palpitations, breathlessness, spoon shaped depression of the nails (koilonychia) and the patient has pallor of the skin. Most symptoms of anaemia occur because the haemoglobin concentration in the blood falls when there is a lack of iron, the red cells become smaller and can carry less oxygen than normal. In this country, where generally people are well fed, anaemia is common and affects between 2-4% of males and at least 10% of the females.

Iron deficiency anaemia occurs for several reasons:
1   Lack of iron in the diet. Many diets are inadequate in their iron content, especially if there is a lack of protein foods in the diet such as meat and eggs.
2   Excessive loss of blood from the body, due to haemorrhage or menstrual loss. The menstrual loss can be averaged out to a loss of 1.2 mg of iron per day in women of child bearing age. There is also a loss of iron in the faeces, sweat, urine, dead skin cells and hair. Normally the body retains as much iron as it possibly can; for example as red cells are broken down most of the iron stays in the body and is reused.
3   Poor absorption of iron. Absorption of iron takes place in the small intestine. Only 10-15% of the iron eaten in the diet is absorbed. Several factors affect iron absorption:
(a)   Vitamin C enhances iron absorption when it is eaten in the diet at

the same time as the iron containing foods.
(b)   Lack of gastric hydrochloric acid generally decreases iron absorption.
(c)   The presence of phytic acid in food inhibits absorption.
(d)   During pregnancy there is an increase in the percentage of iron absorbed from the diet.
(e)   The chemical form of the dietary iron. The ferrous form of iron is absorbed better than the ferric form.
(f)   A person suffering from iron deficiency anaemia can usually absorb a higher percentage of iron from the diet than a healthy person.
(g)   The state of the bone marrow and the amount of iron in the iron stores also affect iron absorption.

The mechanism of iron absorption in the small intestine is extremely complex. After the iron has been absorbed some is taken to the bone marrow for the production of red blood corpuscles, some is used by the cells for the manufacture of enzymes, the remainder is stored in the liver, spleen and bone marrow as the iron-protein compounds ferritin and haemosiderin. Iron deficiency anaemia can be treated with iron rich foods and also various ferrous salts can be administered which are cheap and effective.

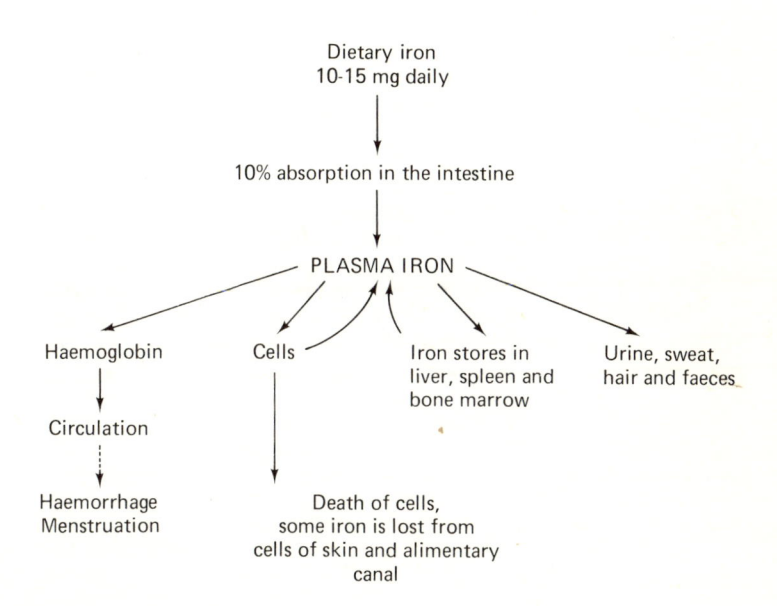

Dietary iron
10-15 mg daily
↓
10% absorption in the intestine
↓
PLASMA IRON

- Haemoglobin → Circulation ⋮ → Haemorrhage, Menstruation
- Cells → Death of cells, some iron is lost from cells of skin and alimentary canal
- Iron stores in liver, spleen and bone marrow
- Urine, sweat, hair and faeces

Minerals and Water

Recommended daily allowance of iron

Girls and boys 15-18 years	15 mg
Men	10 mg
Women 18-55 years	12 mg
Women 55 yrs and over	10 mg
Pregnant and nursing mothers	15 mg

Babies are born with a reserve supply of iron amounting to 200-400 mg. This iron is very important as neither the mother's milk nor cow's milk contains sufficient iron for the baby. The reserve supply of iron should last the baby until it is weaned on to iron containing foods such as egg yolk, cereals and broth.

Food sources of iron

In this country one third of our dietary iron comes from cereals. All white flour is enriched with iron, so bread, cakes and biscuits provide us with iron. A further one third of our iron comes from meat and one sixth comes from vegetables. The iron content of vegetables varies enormously with iron content of the soil.

Iron content of 100 g portions of food

mg of iron per 100 g of food		mg of iron per 100 g of food	
Curry powder	75.00	Egg	2.53
Liver, ox, fried	20.70	Bread, brown	2.44
Ground ginger	17.20	Boiled lentils	2.20
Bovril	12.10	Baked beans	2.05
Corned beef	9.80	Peaches, canned	1.93
Black treacle	9.17	Herring, fried	1.90
Liquorice Allsorts	8.05	Sultanas	1.82
Parsley	8.00	Bread, white	1.80
Beef, steak, fried	6.00	Pears, canned	1.75
Mustard and cress	4.54	Watercress	1.62
Almonds	4.23	Dried apricots, stewed	1.36
Desiccated coconut	3.59	Potatoes cooked in jackets	0.90
Plain chocolates	2.90	Red wine	0.3-1.3
Bacon, back, fried	2.80	Cheddar cheese	0.57
Loganberries, canned	2.88	Butter	0.16
Chicken, roast	2.60	Milk	0.08

Trace Elements

Food portions supplying 12 mg of iron (the daily allowance)

	mg of iron
1 egg, 56 g	1.30
4 slices of bread, white, 100 g	1.80
100 g of beef steak	4.30
50 g of cooked greens	0.65
50 g boiled potatoes	0.24
50 g of plain chocolate	1.45
50 g of canned pears	0.87
50 g of bacon, back, fried	1.40
	12.01

Effects of cooking on iron
In common with the rest of the minerals, iron is not destroyed by cooking. Some iron can leach into the cooking water. If vegetables are prepared and then soaked in water some iron can be lost. It is possible to increase the iron content of foods by cooking in iron pots.

Effects of an excess iron intake
Accidental poisoning of children with iron tablets can occur. Disease of the liver can occur if there is an excessive intake of iron or if a higher percentage of iron is absorbed from the intestine than usual.

TRACE ELEMENTS

IODINE
The body contains 20-50 mg of iodine, 10 mg are present in the thyroid gland. Iodine is found in sea water and has been used as an antiseptic for many years. In 1820 iodine was first used to cure goitre in Switzerland.

Functions of iodine in the body
Iodine is quickly absorbed from food and water in small intestine and passes into the circulation. The thyroid gland absorbs a proportion of this iodine and uses it to make its hormone, thyroxine. Thyroxine plays a part in the control of the rate of metabolism in the body.

Signs of deficiency of iodine
The thyroid gland swells up and gives rise to goitre. It must be mentioned that there are other factors besides iodine deficiency which help to cause goitre. Apart from a swelling of the neck there is usually a retardation of the Basal Metabolic Rate and the subject generally becomes slow mentally and physically. Goitre is an endemic disease which occurs in areas away from the sea where the soil is low in its

Minerals and Water

iodine content and therefore the food grown on the soil will be a poor source of iodine. Examples of areas where goitre is endemic are found in the Himalayas, Alps, Pyrenees and the Rocky Mountains.

If a foetus has an inadequate supply of iodine it is born a cretin and it will not develop properly unless iodine is rapidly administered.

Iodine intake can be increased to prevent or treat goitre by eating seafood, using iodised salt and in severe cases thyroxine can be given.

Daily allowances of iodine
150 microgrammes for adults.

Food sources of iodine
Some iodine is present in drinking water in most areas. The amount of iodine present in foods varies with the iodine content of the soil where the food was grown. Vegetation grown on soil near the sea will be a good source of iodine. Usually if sea fish is eaten at one or two meals per week this provides a daily intake of iodine of over 150 microgrammes.

	Microgrammes per 100 g
Seaweed	4800
Haddock	659
Sardines	36
Herrings	21-27
Eggs	9.4
Spinach	4.8
Milk	2.0
White bread	0.2

There are substances called goitrogens in some foods which prevent the absorption of iodine. They are found in kale, Brussels sprouts and soya beans but their effect in a mixed diet is a very slight.

FLUORINE

Fluorine is found in all tissues of the body especially in the bones and teeth. Fluorine containing minerals are widely distributed in nature and consequently some fluorine is present in natural water.

Functions of fluorine in the body
Fluorine hardens the teeth enamel making teeth more resistant to decay.

Signs of deficiency of fluorine
In a population where there is a very small amount of fluorine in the water there is a high incidence of dental caries. Excess fluorine results in a mottling of the teeth.

Daily allowance of fluorine
The requirement for fluorine is not really known, most adults ingest 2-3 mg per day. Only 5-10% of fluorine in food is absorbed.

Food sources of fluorine
Sea fish contain 5-10 parts per million.
Tea, dry, contains up to 100 parts per million.
Hard waters can contain over 10 parts per million. Soft waters may be free of fluorine. There is less dental decay where there is at least 1 part per million.

COPPER
All tissues of the body contain small amounts of copper. The total weight of copper in the body is 100-150 mg; this being found mainly in muscle and bones.

Functions of copper in the body
Formation of enzymes.

Signs of deficiency of copper
Deficiency of copper is not seen in man.

Daily allowance of copper
A normal diet contains about 2 mg of copper and this seems to be adequate.

Food sources of copper
Copper tends to follow iron distribution in foods. It is found in liver, kidney, green vegetables and chocolate.

COBALT
Cobalt is of interest in as much as it must be provided in the diet as part of vitamin B12.

ZINC
There are 1-2 g of zinc in the body, mainly in the red blood cells, eyes, nails and hair.

Functions of zinc in the body
1 Enzyme synthesis.
2 Zinc is probably concerned with growth and maturation of the human body.

Signs of deficiency of zinc
Zinc deficiency has not been clearly demonstrated in man.

Minerals and Water

Food sources of zinc
Oysters, sea fish, beef, liver, chicken, cornflakes, peas, egg yolk and potatoes.

PRACTICAL WORK ON MINERALS

1   Weigh all food eaten for several days. Using food tables calculate your average daily iron and calcium intakes and compare with recommended allowances.
2   Set out 1 tray showing foods which would provide the daily iron allowance for a pregnant woman and 1 tray showing foods which would provide the daily calcium allowance for a boy aged 18 years.

WATER

The role of water in nutrition
Water is the most important and widely used raw material of all. It is vital to animal, human and plant nutrition. In nutrition, water is not just a solvent, but it takes part in the hydrolysis of proteins, fats and carbohydrates. It provides a vehicle for the transport of raw materials, waste products and the heat liberated by chemical action. Water has special roles in the body in that it helps to lubricate joints, it is found in the cerebrospinal fluid, in the eye and the ear.
Water makes up approximately two-thirds of the human body. In order to keep the quantity of water in the body constant a balance must be maintained between the water loss and the water gain.

Daily gain	*ml*	*Daily loss*	*ml*
Drinking	1300	Evaporation from lungs	400
Food	850	Evaporation from skin	500
Food oxidation	350	Water in urine	1500
		Water in faeces	100
	2500		2500

Water is supplied to the body in the fluids that are drunk, from solid food and water is obtained from the oxidation of protein, fat and carbohydrate. A minimum of 1300 ml should be drunk per day. A diet of 3000 Calories when oxidised in the body will provide 350 ml of water.
Water is lost from the body from the lungs, skin, kidneys and

Minerals

Name	Uses in the body	Deficiency signs	Sources	Recommended daily allowance
Sodium	Nerve conduction Maintenance of acid-base balance	Miner's cramp	Cheese, bacon, ham kippers	0.5 g
Potassium	Nerve conduction Maintenance of acid-base balance	Muscular weakness	Meat, milk, vegetables, cereals, nuts	
Calcium	Bone and tooth formation Blood clotting	Rickets, osteomalcia tetany	Milk, cheese, nuts, green vegetables, bread	500 mg
Phosphorus	Metabolism Bone and tooth formation	Not known in man	Meat, milk, eggs, cheese, nuts, fish, green vegetables	
Iron	Formation of haemoglobin and myoglobin	Iron deficiency anaemia	Liver, cocoa, meat, eggs, curry, green vegetables, bread	10–12 mg
Iodine	Formation of thyroxine in the thyroid gland	Goitre	Sea foods. Eggs, vegetables and cereals	150 μg
Fluorine	Prevention of tooth decay	Tooth decay	Drinking water, sea foods, tea	
Copper	Enzyme formation	Not shown in man	Liver, kidney, green vegetables, chocolate	
Zinc	Enzyme synthesis	Poor growth rate	Sea food, meat, cereals, vegetables	

Minerals and Water

intestine. The loss of water from the skin varies tremendously with the external temperature. In hot climates more than 10 litres of sweat can be lost per day. The loss of water from the body varies with the amount of fluid taken in either in liquid or solid food form. Gut losses of water vary with the type of diet; water loss increases as the level of roughage intake increases.

The amount of water in the body at any instance is regulated by the sensation of thirst and by the antidiuretic hormone which can delay loss of water through the kidneys if it is necessary for the body to retain water.

Babies have a larger turnover of water than adults, in proportion to their body weight. They lose more water through their lungs, skin and kidneys per kilogramme body weight than an adult. More water is lost through a baby's skin because of the relatively large body surface area. Babies are unable to concentrate urine as much as adults and so they require more water to excrete the same amount of nitrogenous waste and mineral salts. Thus a baby's fluid intake must be higher than that of an adult per kilogramme otherwise signs of dehydration appear.

Three days without water is enough to alter a subject's appearance and behaviour and the volume of the body fluid goes down by 10%. In starvation water is more important than solid food.

% water content of some common foods

Butter	13.9	Potatoes, old, boiled	80.5
Cheese	37.0	Apples	84.1
Bread	38.3	Oranges, flesh only	86.1
Beef, lean	68.3	Milk	87.0
Bananas	70.7	Tomatoes	93.4
Eggs	73.4	Cabbage, boiled	95.0
Cod	79.2	Beans, french, boiled	95.5
Peas, boiled	80.0	Marrow, boiled	97.8

7
Milk

Composition of cow's milk

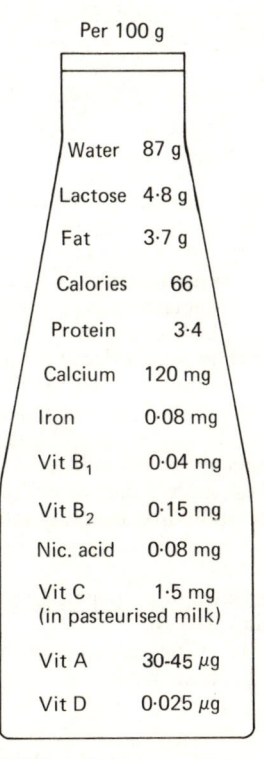

	Per 100 g
Water	87 g
Lactose	4·8 g
Fat	3·7 g
Calories	66
Protein	3·4
Calcium	120 mg
Iron	0·08 mg
Vit B_1	0·04 mg
Vit B_2	0·15 mg
Nic. acid	0·08 mg
Vit C (in pasteurised milk)	1·5 mg
Vit A	30–45 µg
Vit D	0·025 µg

The vitamin A and D content of milk varies with the time of year. Milk is a nutritious food providing most of the nutrients that are necessary for health. Unfortunately some of these nutrients are not present in adequate quantities, especially iron and vitamin C. A baby is

Milk

born with reserve supplies of iron in its liver which will last for 3-5 months, and this prevents iron deficiency anaemia if milk is the sole article in the diet. Usually the baby is weaned on to iron containing foods before the reserve supply of iron has run out. A supplement of vitamin C can be added to the baby's diet in the form of orange or blackcurrant juice or rosehip syrup.

Milk is an example of an oil in water emulsion. This can easily be seen if a drop of milk is placed on a microscope slide, a coverslip put over it, and the slide is examined under the microscope.

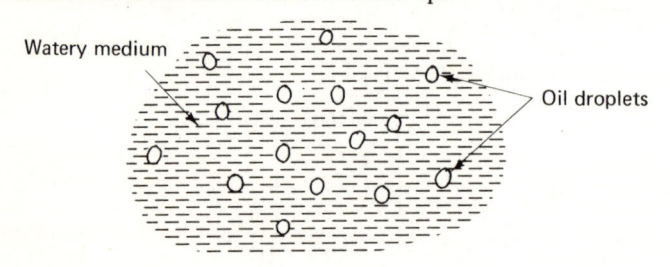

The fat in milk is highly emulsified, making milk easily digested. The emulsifiers in milk are lecithin and protein.

The protein content of milk is as follows:

      Caseinogen 2.6%
      Lactalbumen 0.5%
      Lactoglobulin 0.3%

The only carbohydrate in milk is lactose (milk sugar), which is only mildly sweet. Obtain a sample of lactose from the laboratory and compare its sweetness with that of glucose and sucrose (cane sugar).

Identification of nutrients present in milk

Dilute a sample of fresh milk, 1 part of milk to 2 parts of water. Add glacial acetic acid to the milk drop by drop until there is a clot floating on a clear solution.

Filter

Dry the precipitate with filter paper. Use the precipitate for the Biuret Test and the Sudan III Test.

Neutralise the filtrate using ammonium hydroxide and use for Mollisch's Test and the Lactosazone Test.

Clotting of milk

At an acid pH the enzyme rennin coagulates milk by converting the caseinogen into casein. The casein reacts with calcium forming a clot. Rennin is present in the gastric juice of infants and it can be purchased in the form of rennet which is extracted from the fourth stomach of calves.

Various Forms of Milk

Fruit juice, salt and tannin in strong tea cause milk to clot.

Heating milk

The two milk proteins lactalbumen and lactoglobulin are coagulated by heat and as milk is heated these form a skin on the top of the milk. As heating continues the skin becomes thicker as more protein coagulates and water evaporates from the surface. Air bubbles in the milk expand when heated and lift up the skin causing the milk to boil over. Milk proteins also tend to coagulate on the inside of the milk saucepan; these form a scum which can cause scorching.

The various forms in which milk can be purchased

Pasteurised

Some raw milk is consumed in this country but 90% of our milk has undergone heat treatment or pasteurisation. This process ensures that pathogenic organisms, such as those causing TB, are destroyed.

The milk is heated to $72°C$ and held for 15 secs and then it is cooled. This process does not affect the flavour of milk but it may cause some loss of vitamins C and B1.

Homogenised

This is milk which has been forced through small holes so that the fat globules are reduced in size by 500 times. There is no cream layer in homogenised milk as the small droplets of fat do not rise to the top of the milk.

Sterilised

This is milk which has been heated to a high temperature so that it is rendered sterile. The flavour of the milk is slightly 'cooked' and there is some loss of heat labile vitamins.

Ultra-High Temperature (UHT) or Long-Life

This milk is processed by heating it to $132°C$ for 1 second. This treatment sterilises the milk and gives it long keeping properties. It will keep for several months without refrigeration. Once opened, however, its keeping qualities are the same as those of pasteurised milk. This milk is useful for campers, climbers and those catering for the air and shipping lines. It is also being used extensively in countries where the local milk supply is inadequate and where temperatures prevent the use of pasteurised milk.

Dried

Milk has a high percentage of water and can be conveniently preserved by drying. This cuts down on the problem of transporting large volumes of water. When reconstituted with water dried milk has a very similar nutritive value to that of pasteurised milk. Dried milks can be made from whole milk or from partially or completely skimmed milk. Dried milk is a very rich source of protein and calcium and can be conveniently added to many dishes to increase their nutritive value.

Milk

Evaporated
This is milk which has been heated to reduce its water content to 68%. The milk is then put into cans, sealed and sterilised. Once the can has been opened the life of the milk is short.

Condensed
This is evaporated milk with sugar added to it. Once the can is opened it has a longer life than evaporated milk as the sugar acts as a preservative. The sugar also increases the energy content of the milk making it unsuitable for infant feeding.

Comparison of nutritive content of milks

per 100 g	Protein g	Fat g	Calories	Calcium mg
Milk, whole	3.4	3.7	66	120
Milk, skimmed	3.5	0.2	35	124
Milk, sweetened, condensed	8.2	12.0	354	344
Milk, evaporated	7.8	8.4	155	290
Milk, dried, whole	27.0	29.7	530	960
Milk, dried, skimmed	34.5	0.3	326	1265
Human milk	2.0	3.7	68	25

EXPERIMENTS

EXPERIMENT 1

Obtain samples of all the different types of milk. Set up tasting panels to compare their flavour. This can be done by using the various types of milk to make tea or coffee. Label the samples A, B, C, D, E, F, etc. Make out a short questionnaire to give to the tasters, eg you are asked to taste the six samples of coffee, each one has been prepared using a different type of milk. When you have tasted all 6 samples please fill in the questionnaire. In order to clear the palate between each sample you are asked to sip some water.

Indicate your answer by ringing, A, B, C, D, E or F in each case.
1 Which sample do you prefer?   A, B, C, D, E, F
2 Which sample do you like least?   A, B, C, D, E, F
3 Which sample is the sweetest?   A, B, C, D, E, F
4 Which sample contains the most fat?   A, B, C, D, E, F

Action of Rennin

EXPERIMENT 2

Using the same milks as in the above experiment, find out the weight of milk used in each case to make a standard cup of tea or coffee, calculate the number of Calories obtained per cup and the cost of the milk per cup.

Type of milk	Wt of milk per cup	Cals per 100 g	Cals per cup	Cost of milk per cup

EXPERIMENT 3

Take the samples of different types of milk. Measure pH of each when fresh, after 2 days, after a week, and after 2 weeks when stored at room temperature. Also note flavour, smell and colour at each stage.

Type of milk	pH when fresh	pH after 2 days	pH after 1 week	pH after 2 weeks	Comments on flavour, smell, and colour

Experiment to illustrate the action of the enzyme rennin in various concentrations

Apparatus
    100 ml measuring cylinder
    5 test tubes in rack
    10 ml pipette
    1 ml graduated pipette
    2 ml graduated pipette
    water bath
    Centigrade thermometer
    Stopwatch

Reagents
    The enzyme rennin, obtained in the form of rennet
    50 ml of fresh milk

Method
Measure 15 ml of rennet in a measuring cylinder and dilute to 100 ml using distilled water. Take 5 test tubes and to each add 10 ml of milk. Incubate all tubes in a water bath at 37°C.

To tube 1 add 0.50 ml of the dilute rennet. Start the stopwatch as soon as the rennet comes into contact with the milk. Shake the tube and replace in the waterbath. Observe the tube for signs of clotting and when particles of curd appear note the time.

Repeat the experiment using the other 4 tubes containing milk adding to each 0.75 ml, 1.0 ml, 1.25 ml and 1.5 ml of rennet respectively. Note the time taken for clotting to occur in each case. Plot a graph of volume of rennet added against time taken for clotting.

Milk

Results

Volume of rennet in ml	Clotting time in minutes
0.50	
0.75	
1.00	
1.25	
1.50	

Conclusion
As would be expected in this experiment the greater the volume of rennet used, the shorter is the clotting time. This illustrates that enzyme action is greatly affected by concentration.

A further experiment could be done to show that enzyme action is greatly affected by the concentration of the substrate, which in this case would be diluted milk.

Experiment to illustrate the optimum temperature for the action of rennin

Apparatus
    10 ml pipette   6 thermometers
    6 test tubes in rack   1 ml graduated pipette
    6 water baths

Reagents
    Fresh milk
    Rennin

Method
Pipette 10 ml of milk into each of 6 test tubes. Incubate 1 tube at each of the following temperatures for 10 minutes:
                30°, 40°, 50°, 60°, 70° and 80°C

Pipette 0.5 ml of rennin (diluted as in the previous experiment) into each test tube in turn noting the clotting time.

Plot a graph of temperature against time taken for clotting to occur to find the optimum temperature for the action of rennin.

8
Milk Products

CREAM

When milk stands, the fat globules rise to the top as these are less dense than the watery phase. This fatty layer or cream can be skimmed off or the milk can be centrifuged, in which case the whey or the watery part of the milk will go to the outside of the centrifuge and the cream goes to the inside.

Cream is an emulsion of milk fat which is high in its Calorie content. It contains small amounts of lactose, protein, B vitamins and vitamin D. It is quite a good source of vitamin A.

Nutrient content of cream per 100 g

	Single cream	Double cream
Calories	219	462
Protein g	2.4	1.5
Fat g	21.2	48.2
Lactose g	3.2	2.0

Soured cream

Soured cream is made from single cream which has a bacterial culture added to it to sour it.

Whipping cream

Whipping quality of cream varies with several factors, the most important being the percentage fat content of the cream. The percentage of fat present should be above 30-35%. Double cream will whip well as it has 48.2% fat; but single cream will not whip as it has only 21.2% fat. The larger fat globules found in Channel Islands cream form a stiffer whip and it whips more readily.

As cream is whipped, the structure becomes more complex. The air bubbles are surrounded by protein films and lumps of fat globules are usually held within the protein films. In whipped cream the fat globules prevent air from escaping. Whipped cream is an air in water foam. Over-whipping results in the formation of butter.

When cream is cold it is stiff but when it is heated the fat melts and the foam collapses.

Milk Products

The best temperature for whipping cream is 4°C as the fat globules are hard at this temperature and give a stiffer whip. The bowl, the whisk and the cream should be kept cold for the best results.

Cream at least 24 hrs old whips better than fresh cream.

Experiment to Prepare Cream
Apparatus
   Glass beakers
   A large shallow spoon
Reagents
   4 pints of milk
Method

Pour the milk into several beakers. Allow to stand for ¼ hour or until there is a definite cream line. Skim off the cream layer carefully using a shallow spoon.

Examine and taste the sample of cream produced.

If separating funnels are available these can be used to separate the milk and the cream.

BUTTER
Nutrient content of butter per 100 g

Calories	793
Protein	0.4 g
Fat	85.1 g
Carbohydrate	Trace
Calcium	15 mg
Iron	0.16 mg
Vitamin A	1050 µg
Vitamin D	1.0 µg

Butter contains 13.9% water and useful quantities of vitamin A and D. The content of vitamins A and D varies with the time of year; in the summer, the cows have more carotene in their diet and this increases the vitamin A content of the butter.

The butter consumption per head in the UK in 1970 was 8.8 kg (19.4 lb), compared with 17.9 kg (39.4 lb) in New Zealand and 2.4 kg (5.2 lb) in the USA. In the USA the margarine market is very large.

The firmness of butter depends on the composition of the milk fat which is influenced by the diet of the animal. The fatty acids found in butter in conjunction with glycerol are oleic, palmitic, stearic, myristic and butyric. Oleic acid is the main component and this causes butter to have a low melting point.

Butter is an emulsion of water in oil and is made by churning cream which is an oil in water emulsion.

There are two main types of butter:

Butter

1   Sweet cream butter. This is produced in New Zealand, Australia and Great Britain. It has a mild flavour as it is made from fresh cream. It has a firm smooth texture.

2   Lactic butter. This is made in France, Denmark and Holland. It is made from cream which has been ripened with lactic acid producing bacteria. It has a stronger flavour than sweet cream butter and it creams easily.

Manufacture of butter

It takes about 10.3 l (18 pints) of milk to produce 454 g (1 lb) of butter or 22857 l (5000 gallons) of milk to produce 1 tonne of butter.

Stage 1   The milk is left to stand, the cream rises to the top and is separated from the milk.

Stage 2   The cream is pasteurised to destroy any pathogenic bacteria. If the cream is to be used for lactic butter a culture of Streptococci is added.

Stage 3   The cream is churned at 40°C for about 40 minutes. During churning the fat globules stick together and form grains of butter.

Stage 4   The butter grains are washed and salted if the butter is to be salted butter.

Stage 5   Excess water and air are removed and the butter is pressed together in blocks.

A new method of butter making is used in some creameries called the *Continuous Method*. The cream is fed into large cylinders continuously where it is churned. The buttermilk is removed and the grains are forced through outlets forming a continuous strip of butter.

Butter is used extensively in cookery. Most people prefer its flavour to that of margarine but nutritionally they are very similar.

Effect of heat on butter

Melted butter is clarified by heating it, allowing the solids to settle and skimming off the butterfat. As butter is heated it turns brown, this is known as *beurre noisette* (hazelnut butter) and is used as a sauce with fish and vegetables. As butter is heated further it becomes dark brown and is called beurre noir. This is used with vinegar or lemon juice and parsley for sauces.

Experiment to Prepare Butter

Apparatus
   Screw top jars
   Muslin
   Glass funnel

Material
   Cream

Milk Products

Method

Place cream in screw top jars. Replace the lid and shake until butter grains appear. Strain the contents of the jar through muslin in a glass funnel placed over a jar. Butter is left on the muslin and the liquid is buttermilk.

Place a smear of the butter produced on a microscope slide and examine under the microscope.

Buttermilk is used for animal feeding and for the production of milk powder.

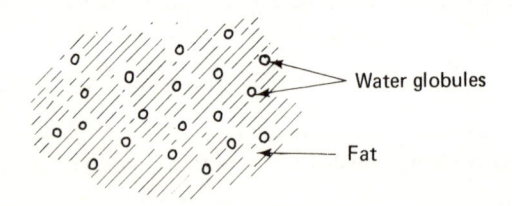

CHEESE

The making of cheese is an old method of preserving milk. During cheese making the nutrients of milk are concentrated so cheese is a highly nutritious food. There are many different types of cheese, their composition varies with the type of milk used, the breed of the animal, the acidity of the milk, the processing techniques and the microorganisms which are used as well as many other factors.

The nutritional value of cheese

The nutritional value of different types of cheese varies considerably.

Per 100 g	Protein g	Fat g	Carbohydrate g	Calories	Calcium mg
Camembert	22.8	23.2	Trace	309	152
Cheddar	25.4	34.5	Trace	425	810
Cream	3.3	86.0	Trace	813	30
Danish Blue	23.0	29.2	Trace	366	578
Edam	24.4	22.9	Trace	313	739
Cottage	19.5	3.9	4	113	81

Cottage cheese is an acid curd cheese made from pasteurised fat-free milk. The curd is cut into small cubes, heated slowly, the whey is drained off and the curd is washed several times and cooled. Salt and single cream are then added. Cottage cheese is useful in reducing diets as it is much lower in Calories due to its low fat content.

Cheese

Cheddar is the commonest type of cheese eaten in this country and consists of roughly one third fat, one third protein, and one third water. It contains 419 µg of vitamin A and 0.35 µg of vitamin D per 100 g.

Cheese is a good source of high quality protein and has a high content of calcium and phosphorus. It contains some of the B vitamins but no vitamin C or carbohydrate and it has a low iron content.

The manufacture of cheddar cheese

Cheddar cheese is a popular hard pressed cheese with long storage properties. The original cheddar cheese was made in Cheddar, Somerset. 10 litres of milk produces 1 kg of cheese.

Stage 1   The milk is pasteurised and pumped into large vats.
Stage 2   A culture of lactic acid producing bacteria is added to the milk to ripen it.
Stage 3   Rennet, which contains the enzyme rennin is added to clot the milk turning it into curds and whey.
Stage 4   When the milk is at the desired level of acidity the curd is cut into cubes to help separate the whey.
Stage 5   The mixture is stirred and heated to 37°C by passing steam through the jacket surrounding the vat. This heating aids the separation of the whey and the curd and improves the texture of the curd.
Stage 6   The whey is run off, the curd is cut. The blocks of curd are piled on top of each other to aid draining.
Stage 7   The blocks of curd are cut into small pieces about the size of a walnut and salt is added using 1 kg of salt per 500 litres of milk. The salt brings out the flavour of the cheese and acts as preservative.
Stage 8   The salted curd is then packed into moulds, pressed to remove any further whey and placed in a ripening room where it is stored for 3 months or more. During storage development of flavour occurs.

Effect of cooking on cheese

When cheese is cooked it softens to become a viscous liquid and some fat tends to separate out. When cheese is overcooked the cheese becomes tough and stringy. High fat cheeses cook better than low fat cheeses. If cheese is grated and the temperature kept low it is much less likely to become stringy on cooking.

Yogurt

Yogurt is a form of fermented milk. It contains all the nutrients of milk except for lactose which is converted to lactic acid by the lactic acid producing bacteria. It is a very useful food in the diet as it is easily digested and thus has a role to play in feeding the elderly and those who are convalescing.

Yogurt is a good source of protein, calcium and phosphorus. It is

Milk Products

thought by many to have certain beneficial properties such as improving intestinal function.

Comparison of nutritional value of natural and fruit yogurt
Per 142 g carton

	Calories	Protein g	Fat g	Calcium mg	Carbohydrate g
Natural, low fat	90	5.6	1.5	200	7.0
Fruit, low fat	120	4.0	1.1	200	15.0

Preparation of yogurt in the laboratory
Yogurt can be made from whole, partially skimmed, evaporated or dried milk.

Method

Heat 100 ml of milk to 80°C for 5-10 mins. Cool to 45°C and then add 2-3 ml of yogurt starter culture. Incubate at 45°C for 3 hours and then transfer to a refrigerator where acidity develops.

Commercially yogurt is made by first homogenising the milk and heating it to 90-100°C and then cooling it to 40-45°C. Then the culture of *Lactobacillus bulgaricus, Streptococcus thermophilus* and *Lactobacillus acidophilus* is added. The yogurt is then kept at 40°C for about 3 hours when the acidity should have developed and clotting takes place. The yogurt is then kept at 4°C until required. Yogurt only has a limited life and should be eaten before too much acidity develops.

Ice cream
Ice cream consists of fat, sugar, stabilisers, colour and flavour. There are two main types of ice cream sold in this country: dairy and non-dairy ice cream.

Both types of ice cream must contain a minimum of 5% fat and 7½% solid non-fat. If ice cream is described as being dairy ice cream all the fat used must be milk fat. Non-dairy ice cream contains vegetable fats such as hydrogenated coconut oil.

Per 100 g

Protein	4.1 g
Fat	11.3 g
Carbohydrate	19.8 g
Calories	196
Calcium	137 mg

9
Eggs

An egg is a unit containing enough food and water for the development of the chick from a single fertilised cell. The chick normally hatches 21 days after the egg is laid.

Eggs are graded according to their weight.

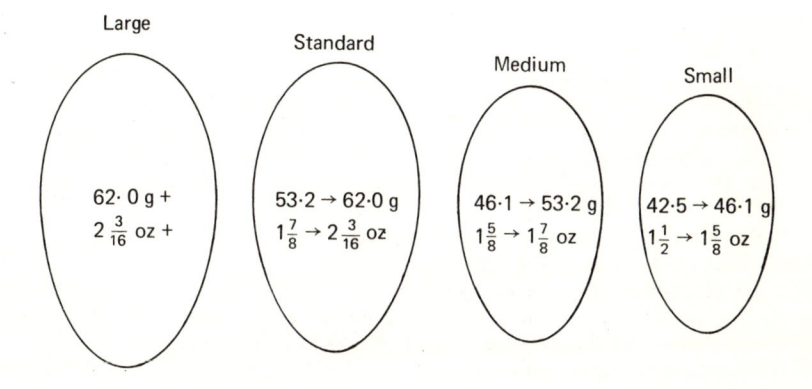

Large	Standard	Medium	Small
62·0 g + $2\frac{3}{16}$ oz +	53·2 → 62·0 g $1\frac{7}{8} \to 2\frac{3}{16}$ oz	46·1 → 53·2 g $1\frac{5}{8} \to 1\frac{7}{8}$ oz	42·5 → 46·1 g $1\frac{1}{2} \to 1\frac{5}{8}$ oz

The egg consists of a shell, a shell membrane, egg white and egg yolk.

Composition of an egg

Weight in grammes

Shell and membrane	7.1
White and yolk	49.7
White	35.5
Yolk	14.2
Total weight of egg	56.8

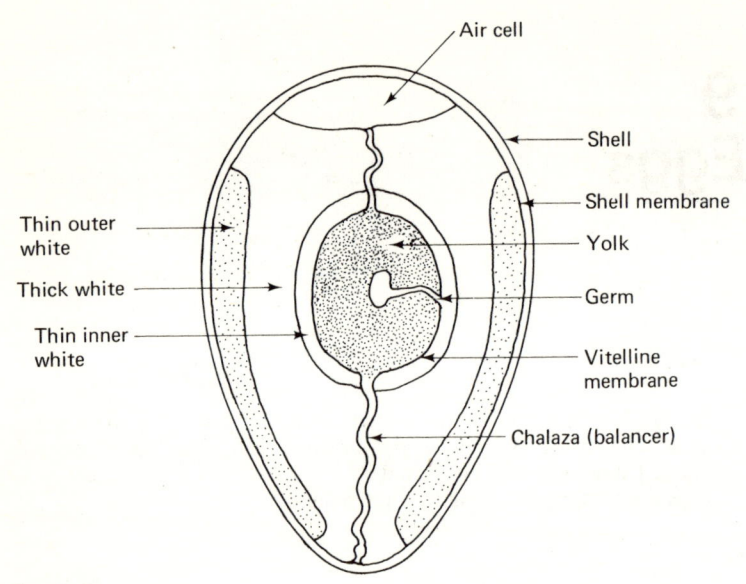

Eggs

Diagram labels: Air cell, Shell, Shell membrane, Yolk, Germ, Vitelline membrane, Chalaza (balancer), Thin outer white, Thick white, Thin inner white

The shell
The shell consists of 97% calcium carbonate and 3% protein and organic matter. It is quite strong as it has to bear the weight of the growing chick. The shell is porous to allow oxygen to reach the chick and carbon dioxide to leave the shell. On the inner layer of the shell are two shell membranes which help to prevent bacteria from the atmosphere passing into the egg. After the egg is laid, it cools and contracts and the two shell membranes separate to form the air cell at the rounded end of the egg.

The colour of the egg shell varies from chocolate brown to white and is due to the pigment porphyrin. The colour of the shell is dependent on the breed of the hen and is not indicative of the nutritional value of the egg. As the egg shell is porous the egg must be stored away from strong smelling foods.

Nutrient content of eggs

per 100 g	Water g	Protein g	Fat g	Calories	Carbo-hydrate g	Iron mg	Calcium mg
Whole egg	73.4	11.9	12.3	163	0	2.53	56
Egg white	88.3	9.0	trace	37	0	0.10	5
Egg yolk	51.0	16.2	30.5	350	0	6.13	131

Egg white

There are two types of white present in the egg, the thin white and the thick white which differ in their physical and chemical properties.

Egg white is an unusual animal tissue in that it has a high percentage of water.

There are nine different types of protein in the egg white, including ovalbumen and conalbumen. A small amount of the protein avidin is present; this combines with biotin, one of the B vitamins, and makes the biotin unavailable to the body. When the egg is cooked avidin is broken down so that the biotin can be used by the body.

Egg white contains vitamins of the B complex and minerals but it does not contain fat or carbohydrate.

Egg yolk

Egg yolk is an emulsion of fat globules dispersed in water, stabilised by lecithin. The egg yolk contains a higher proportion of protein than the white and a lower proportion of water. The proteins present are simple proteins called livetins and complex proteins called phosphoproteins. Egg yolk has a high fat content, ie 30.5%. The fat contains the fat soluble vitamins A, D, E and K. The colour of the yolk is not indicative of nutritional value. The yolk contains some minerals notably iron and the B vitamins. The carotene content of the yolk varies with the diet of the hen. Unfortunately, egg yolk is exceptionally high in its cholesterol content. This means that people on a low cholesterol diet often have to cut down their intake of eggs to 1 or 2 per week.

Apart from the cholesterol problem eggs are an excellent food providing protein of the highest quality and a good range of vitamins and minerals. In the days of high food prices eggs provide a rich source of protein at moderate cost.

Chalazae

There are two chalazae or balancers in the egg which hold the yolk in position. During storage the chalazae become weaker and the yolk tends to move towards the shell making it vulnerable to bacteria passing through the shell. If the egg is stored correctly with the air cell upwards the air cell acts as a barrier between the yolk and the bacteria in the atmosphere.

Changes which occur in the egg during storage

Eggs should not be washed before storage as this removes the slimy mucin which is on the outside of the shell. The mucin decreases the porosity of the shell. The changes which occur during storage are minimised if the eggs are kept at a low temperature.

As eggs are stored water vapour is lost through the shell and consequently the liquid part of the egg decreases in size and the air cell gets larger. Carbon dioxide tends to be lost through the shell and as a result

Eggs

the pH of the white increases, ie the egg white becomes more alkaline. There is a movement of water inside the egg between the white and the yolk through the vitelline membrane. This movement takes place by osmosis. The yolk has a higher osmotic pressure than the white and the vitelline membrane is semi-permeable. Water therefore moves from the white to the yolk from the region of lower concentration to the region of higher concentration. The vitelline membrane stretches as the yolk increases in size and after a time the vitelline membrane breaks and the white and the yolk mix.

Movement of water from the white to the yolk by osmosis

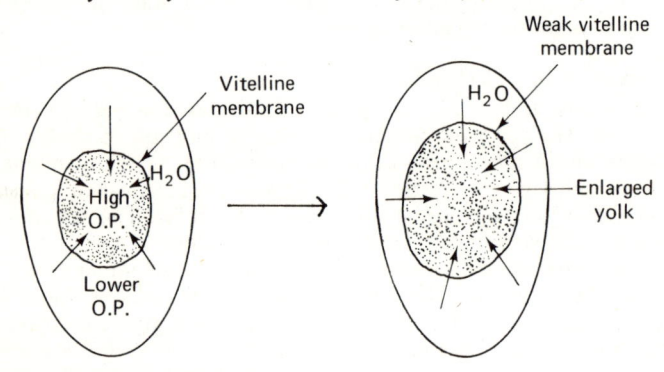

During storage the thick white becomes thinner and the chalazae weaken.

Characteristics of a fresh egg
1 The vitelline membrane is intact.
2 The pH of the white is about 7.9.
3 When cracked the thick white should support the yolk and should be thick.

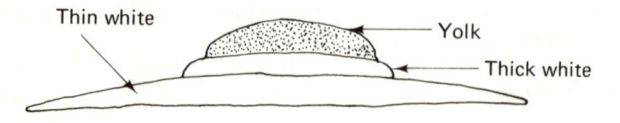

4 When a fresh egg is cooked the white is curdy and very white in colour.

Characteristics of a stale egg
1 The vitelline membrane is weak and so when a stale egg is cracked the yolk usually mixes with the white. If the egg is very stale the vitelline membrane breaks in the intact egg.

2   The pH of the white is about 9.3.
3   When cracked the thick white has become thin so that it does not support the yolk and the egg spreads out further than a fresh egg.

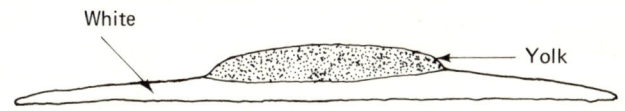

```
         White
           ↓
    ╭──────────────╮
   ╱   ░░░░░░░░    ╲  ←— Yolk
  ╱_____╲
```

4   When a stale egg is cooked the white has a greyish-yellow tinge and has a very firm consistency.

Methods used to preserve eggs
1   *Drying*
Eggs can be conveniently preserved by spray or roller drying. Some eggs are preserved by the Accelerated Freeze Drying (AFD) process. Dried eggs can be reconstituted with water. They are used in the catering and food industries.
2   *Freezing*
The white and the yolk of the eggs are mixed and then the mixture is pasteurised to eliminate pathogenic bacteria. The eggs are then frozen and stored in tins. Frozen eggs are used in flour confectionary.
3   *Water glass*
Eggs can be stored for long periods if they are immersed in water glass. The water glass prevents movement of gases and bacteria through the shell. This method of egg preservation was used extensively during the last war when egg supplies were unreliable.
4   *Gas storage*
If eggs are stored in 2.5% carbon dioxide losses of carbon dioxide from the egg are reduced and so the pH changes which affect the structure of the egg are minimised.
5   *Cold storage*
If eggs are stored at a low temperature, the humidity of the atmosphere can be increased to decrease evaporation through the shell. The low temperature decreases the growth rate of moulds making it possible to increase the humidity.
6   *Oil dipping*
Eggs can be dipped in a light oil and this decreases the porosity of the shell to gases and bacteria.

Discolouration of yolk after hard boiling
A hard boiled egg usually has a bluish-black discoloration at the junction of the white and the yolk. This colour is due to the formation of ferrous sulphide which may be formed from the interaction of iron in the yolk and sulphur in the white. This discoloration is prevented if the egg is rapidly cooled in cold running water immediately after cooking, as this draws the gases away from the junction.

Effect of cooking on eggs

As eggs are cooked the white and yolk colloids change from liquids into solids in the process called coagulation. The egg white changes from a clear liquid to a white opaque solid at about 62°C. The yolk reaches the stage when it is solid between 65° and 70°C. Heat is absorbed during coagulation of egg proteins so the reaction is said to be endothermic. When egg custard is made as the custard thickens the temperature remains the same or even falls. Coagulation temperature depends on cooking temperature, the presence of water, acid, sugar, salt, etc.

The proteins in eggs are present as globular shaped coils which are held in place by weak chemical bridges. During some cooking methods the protein is denatured, eg during heating and also egg white beating, this means that the chemical bridges are broken, the peptide chains unfold and new bridges can be formed.

Uses of eggs in cookery

1 Eggs are extensively used on their own as boiled, poached or fried eggs.
2 Eggs can be beaten up with milk, cooked in fat and served as scrambled egg. The addition of milk to egg dilutes the protein, raises the temperature at which coagulation occurs and usually weakens the gel.
3 Eggs can be beaten with or without the addition of milk or water and fried to make an omelette.
4 Egg custard. The success of an egg custard depends on obtaining just the right degree of coagulation of the egg. Coagulation of egg custard is affected by temperature, length of cooking and the amount of milk and sugar added. The temperature of a stirred egg custard should be kept below boiling point otherwise it will curdle. Once the egg has coagulated heating must be stopped. The addition of sugar raises the coagulation temperature. If the proportion of egg in the recipe for an egg custard is increased then the coagulation temperature is lowered. If the egg custard is made with more egg white than yolk the custard will coagulate at a lower temperature than usual as egg whites have a lower coagulation temperature than egg yolks.
5 Egg white foam is an important leavening agent in meringues, soufflés and some flour mixtures. Egg white foam is an example of a colloid. It consists of bubbles of air surrounded by egg white protein that has been stretched and dried by the beating process. As egg white is whipped, the enclosed air bubbles become smaller and the colour changes from pale yellow to opaque white, the stiffness and the volume increases. Maximum stability of the foam is achieved before maximum volume. Overbeating causes the volume and stability to decrease, too much air is trapped and the albumen stretches too much becoming

inelastic and releasing liquid. The properties of egg white foams that are of interest are stiffness, volume, texture and stability. Slightly beaten egg white foams are used for clarifying soups and as thickening agents. Egg white foams at the wet peak stage, when the foam will flow, are used for soft meringues. Egg white foams at the stiff peak stage, when air cells are very small, are used for omelettes, soufflés and meringues.

Effect of various agents on egg white foam
(a) Temperature   Egg whites at refrigerator temperatures beat more slowly than those at room temperature.
(b) Sugar   Sugar retards the denaturation of the egg white and so slows down foam formation but the addition of sugar makes a smoother more stable foam.
(c) Acids, eg citric acid in lemon juice. Acids seem to increase the beating time required to make a foam and also increase the stability of the foam.
(d) Water, milk, egg yolk and oils. All these generally seem to decrease foam stability and volume.
(e) Salt   Salt decreases the volume and stability of the foam if the foam is beaten for a short time.
6   Eggs are used for binding and coating croquettes, fish cakes etc.
7   In baked goods eggs are able to hold ingredients in the meshwork formed when they coagulate on heating.
8   Eggs are used as emulsifying agents in some foods, eg mayonnaise. Vinegar and oil form an emulsion but it is only a temporary emulsion and on standing the oil droplets combine together and separate out. Lecithin, a phospholipid, present in egg yolk, acts as a stabilizing agent in mayonnaise. Lecithin is made of complicated molecules, part of each molecule has an affinity for water and part of it is water hating. The molecule of lecithin can be represented diagrammatically thus:

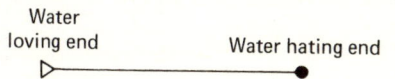

```
       Water
    loving end              Water hating end
       ▷────────────────────────●
```

These molecules of lecithin orientate themselves around the oil globules in mayonnaise and form a protective layer preventing the oil drops from coalescing.

```
                    Lecithin molecule
                         ↓
              (diagram of oil globule with
               lecithin molecules arranged
               around it)
                    ← Oil globule
```

9   Eggs also contribute to the flavour, colour and nutritive value of dishes in which they are used.

EXPERIMENTS WITH EGGS

Set aside 6 eggs at room temperature for a few weeks to provide stale egg samples.

EXPERIMENT 1
Method
Weigh 1 standard egg. Crack the egg on to a flat surface marked with concentric rings. Note how far the egg spreads, note also odour and appearance of the egg. Weigh the shell, separate white from yolk and weigh each. Measure pH of the white and yolk separately and pH of yolk and white mixed. Repeat the experiment with a stale egg and compare results.

	Fresh egg	Stale egg
Extent of spread on concentric rings in cm		
Odour		
Appearance		
Weight of shell g		
Weight of yolk g		
Weight of white g		
pH of yolk		
pH of white		
pH of yolk + white		

EXPERIMENT 2

Examination of intact eggs for freshness
Method
Dissolve 100 g of salt in 500 ml water in a jug. Lower a fresh egg into the saline. Note the position of the egg. Repeat with a slightly stale egg and a very stale egg.
Results
The fresh egg positions itself on its side in the saline.
The slightly stale egg remains submerged in the saline with its blunt end uppermost.
The very stale egg floats on the saline with its blunt end upwards.

Practical Work

As the egg becomes stale the air cell increases in size and acts as a float. In the fresh egg the size of the air cell is too small to affect the position of the egg in the saline.

EXPERIMENT 3

Experiment to compare the appearance, colour and texture of fresh and stale eggs after boiling
Method
Boil a fresh egg, a slightly stale egg and a very stale egg for 4 minutes. Examine each egg for its appearance, colour and texture.

EXPERIMENT 4

Experiment to determine the coagulation temperature of eggs
Method
Place a beaten fresh egg in a large test tube in a water bath. Heat gently and note the temperature at which the egg coagulates. Repeat using just the white and then just the yolk.
Add some milk to another beaten egg and note the difference in the coagulation temperature. Sugar and salt can also be added to an egg to see their effect on coagulation temperature.

EXPERIMENT 5

Experiment to show the function of eggs in cake mixes
Method
1 Prepare a sponge cake using a standard method and recipe.
2 Prepare the sponge as above but omit the eggs, milk should be used to obtain the correct degree of moisture.
3 Prepare a small fruit cake using a standard method and recipe.
4 Prepare a fruit cake as above but omit the eggs and use milk to make the mixture moist.
Comment on the flavour, texture, crust, colour, etc, of each cake.

EXPERIMENTS ON EGG WHITE FOAMING

EXPERIMENT 1.

To show the effect of temperature on the foaming capacity of egg white
Method
Place egg whites from standard eggs in the following conditions
1 In the refrigerator at $4°C$
2 In a waterbath at $10°C$
3 In a waterbath at $15°C$

Eggs

4 In a waterbath at 20°C
5 In a waterbath at 25°C
6 In a waterbath at 30°C

Whisk each egg white in turn using the same size bowl and the same type of whisk. Measure the time taken to reach the first peak in each case.

At which temperature is the first peak stage reached most readily?

EXPERIMENT 2

To show the effect of degree of freshness on the foaming capacity of egg white
Method
  Obtain the following egg samples
1 1 newly laid egg
2 1 egg 1 week old
3 1 egg 2 weeks old
4 1 egg 3 weeks old
5 1 egg 6 weeks old

Whisk egg white from each egg sample measuring the time taken for the formation of the first peak stage. Does a fresh egg or a stale egg whisk most readily?

EXPERIMENT 3

Experiment to show the microscopic structure of egg white foam at various stages during its preparation
Method
  Whisk 1 fresh egg white to the over-whisked stage. Remove a sample of the foam on to a microscope slide at various stages. Draw the microscopic appearance of the foam.

EXPERIMENT 4

Experiment to determine the stability of an egg white foam at various stages during beating
  The stability of an egg white foam can be conveniently ascertained by measuring the time taken for a certain volume of liquid to leak away from a known weight of foam.
Method
  Beat 3 egg whites and before the first peak stage is reached withdraw 10 g of foam into a preweighed beaker. Place foam in a glass funnel placed over a measuring cylinder. Place a glass plate over the top of the funnel. Measure the time taken for 3 ml of liquid to drip from the foam into the measuring cylinder.

Practical Work

```
           Glass funnel
           Egg white foam




           Measuring cylinder






           Liquid egg white
```

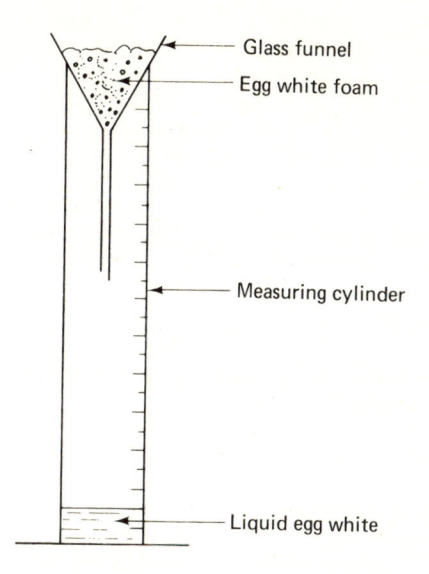

Continue beating the egg white to the first peak stage, and remove 10 g of foam and test for stability. Continue beating and measure stability when the egg white is overbeaten.
Results

Stage	Time taken to collect 3 ml of liquid

EXPERIMENT 5

Experiment to show the effect of certain substances on the stability of egg white foams
Method
 Whisk 3 egg whites to the stage that was found to be most stable in previous experiment. Remove 9,10 g samples and make the following additions.
1 To sample 1 add 1 ml of oil
2 To sample 2 add 1 ml of egg yolk
3 To sample 3 add 1 ml of water

109

Eggs

4   To sample 4 add 0.5 g of salt
5   To sample 5 add 0.5 of sugar
6   To sample 6 add 1 g of sugar
7   To sample 7 add 0.5 g of citric acid
8   To sample 8 add 1 ml of lemon juice
9   To sample 9 add 0.5 g of cream of tartar

    Place each sample in a glass funnel and measure the time taken to collect 3 ml of liquid in each case. Note which substances increase and which substances decrease the stability of the foam.

EXPERIMENT 6

Experiment to show the emulsifying action of egg yolk in the preparation of mayonnaise
Recipe
    142 ml of oil stained with an oil soluble stain
    1 egg yolk
    1 tablespoon of vinegar
    ¼ teaspoon of mustard

    Prepare mayonnaise using the above recipe and remove a few drops of the mixture on to a microscope slide at 3 different stages during the mixing. Observe the 3 slides under the microscope noting the evenness in the structure of mayonnaise when preparation is complete.

    Repeat experiment omitting the egg yolk. In this experiment there will be no lecithin to act as the emulsifying agent so a temporary emulsion is formed.

EXPERIMENT 7

Experiment to determine the effect of adding certain ingredients to an egg custard sauce
Recipe
    2 eggs   28 g sugar
    284 ml milk   Pinch of salt
Method
    Place eggs, sugar and salt in a basin and mix, gradually whisk in the milk. Place in double boiler pan, heat water in boiler to $60°C$ and place pan containing custard mixture over the water. Start stop clock and stir. Heat very slowly and note temperature at which coagulation occurs and time taken to reach the coagulation point. Continue heating and noting the temperature after coagulation has occurred.

    Repeat the experiment using
1   4 egg whites instead of 2 eggs
2   4 egg yolks

Practical Work

3   1 egg only
4   56 g of sugar instead of 28 g
5   Water in place of milk
6   Add 2 teaspoonsful of lemon juice
 Note time taken to reach coagulation point, the coagulation temperature and the consistency of the custard in each case..

10
Meat, Poultry and Fish

Meat consists of the muscle, fat, connective tissue and offals of many species of animals and birds. Meat is not essential in the diet. The amount of meat that is eaten usually depends on income. Poultry includes chicken, turkeys, ducks and geese. The flesh of poultry is very similar to that of animal tissue, containing 20-30% protein.

THE STRUCTURE OF MEAT

Muscle tissue consists of bundles of muscle fibres. Each fibre is surrounded by a layer of connective tissue which is called the endomysium. The muscle fibres lie parallel to one another. The bundles of muscle fibres are surrounded by connective tissue called the perimysium.

Longitudinal section of meat fibres

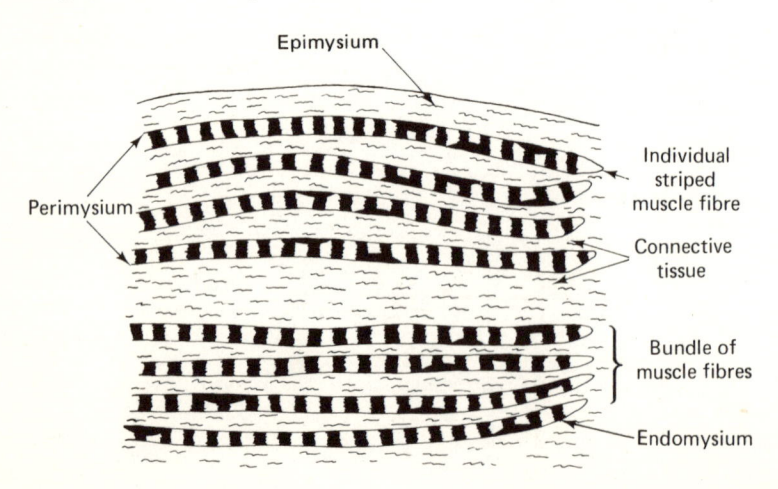

The Structure of Meat

A muscle fibre is spindle shaped and up to 50 mm long and 0.1 m in diameter. In young animals the muscle fibres are slender and these give rise to tender meat. Tough meat can be made more tender by beating it to break down the fibres and by adding an acid, eg lemon juice or vinegar. The connective tissue surrounding the muscle bundles joins on to tendons which attach the muscle to the bone. Blood vessels, nerves and fat cells are embedded in the connective tissue.

The muscle cells contain the proteins actin, myosin, albumen, globulin and the muscle pigment myoglobin. The cells also contain the mineral salts, the B vitamins, fats, carbohydrates, and 78% water. While the animal is alive the carbohydrate in the muscle is glycogen.

The main pigment in meat is myoglobin which is red but on exposure to air the brownish-red pigment metmyoglobin is formed.

Connective tissue

This is responsible for the toughness of meat. The yellow connective tissue contains a high percentage of the substance elastin; and the white connective tissue contains a high percentage of collagen. The connective tissue is composed of small cells. Tendons are mainly made of white connective tissue and ligaments are mainly composed of yellow connective tissue.

The white collagen is non-elastic and very strong and when cooked it softens to form gelatine. The yellow elastin is very resistant to heat and does not soften.

Bones, cartilage and adipose tissue are all connective tissues.

Fat tissue

Fat tissue is made of fatty cells which enlarge as the animal gets fat. Fat is first deposited round the internal organs, eg the heart and kidneys, and then subcutaneously. Fat is next deposited between the muscles and then intramuscularly. The intramuscular fat produces the marbling of meat which improves the flavour and juiciness of meat.

The colour of the fat is due to carotenoids. Lamb and pork have little colour in the fat and beef fat is a pale yellow. The colour of the fat in a cut of meat depends on the age of the animal, its diet and the part of the carcass used.

Post mortem changes

When the animal is alive the muscles should contain glycogen which is the form in which glucose is stored as a reserve supply of energy. When the animal dies glycogen is converted into lactic acid as the metabolism of the muscle cells continues in the absence of oxygen. The lactic acid helps to preserve the meat and decreases the likelihood of infection during storage. The muscle fibres as they have become acid in respect to the body fluid tend to take up water from the body fluids and swell up in rigor mortis.

Meat, Poultry and Fish

If the animal has been starved or exercised before it is killed the glycogen reserves have been used up and therefore no lactic acid develops in the meat. The meat is then flabby and liable to infection.

Enzymes in meat survive after the animal has been killed. The proteolytic enzymes break down the protein and have the effect of tenderising the meat while it is hung. Meat can be tenderised artificially with the enzyme papain.

The cooking of meat

When meat is cooked it should be treated so that it is tender and juicy, it should have a brown surface and there should be a minimal amount of shrinkage. Shrinkage can occur when meat is cooked due to denaturation of proteins and evaporative losses.

The cooking process begins at 60°C and the meat proteins coagulate at 70°C. The muscle fibres tend to shrink and come away from the bone. Extractives are formed. The quantity of extractives formed varies with the age of the animal, the older the animal the more extractives are formed. Veal produces few extractives and therefore has a mild flavour. Extractives contain amino acids, gelatine, minerals, B vitamins and fat.

Summary of the changes which occur on cooking meat

1. The collagen changes into gelatine.
2. The actin and myosin are converted into actomysin.

    ACTIN + MYOSIN = ACTOMYOSIN

3. Extractives are formed.
4. Bacteria are killed.
5. Fat melts and disperses.
6. Digestibility is increased.
7. Some B vitamins are broken down by the heat.
8. The colour changes.

Nutritional value of meat

The consumption of the three main carcass meats in the latter part of 1973 per head per week was 13 oz (369 g), the corresponding figure for poultry was 6.7 oz (190 g).

Household food consumption of some common protein foods expressed as oz per person per week

Beef and veal	6.9	Fish	5.05
Mutton and lamb	4.96	Eggs	8.48
Pork	3.10		
Bacon and ham	4.68	Figures from *Household Food*	
Poultry (uncooked)	5.46	*Consumption and Expenditure 1972*	

Protein
The protein content of meat is high and the protein present is of high biological value.
Fat
The fat content of meat varies with the cut and the diet of the animal. The fat contains a high proportion of saturated fatty acids although this proportion can be modified by changing the fat content of the animal's diet.
Minerals
Meat is a good source of iron and phosphorus but a poor source of calcium.

Vitamins

Vitamin A
Vitamin A. This found in liver, heart and kidneys but only a trace is found in muscle meat.

Vitamin B complex
Meat is a good source of thiamine, nicotinic acid and B12.

Vitamin C
Fresh meat contains a small amount of vitamin C, just enough to prevent scurvy if meat is the sole food in the diet.

Vitamin D
This is found in liver but only a trace is present in muscle meat.

Gelatine

This is obtained commercially from the bones of mature cattle. It is used in food preparation for setting sweet and savoury jellies and in many cold sweets made with milk, eggs, fruit and cream. The food value of gelatine is limited as it contains only 2 of the 8 essential amino acids. In food preparation it takes part in reversible (physical) changes.

Meat, Poultry and Fish

Nutritional value of meat per 100 g edible portion

	Protein g	Fat g	Calories	Calcium mg	Iron mg
Bacon, back, fried	24.6	53.4	597	11.5	2.8
Beef, topside, lean and fat, roast	24.2	23.8	321	5.9	4.4
Chicken, roast	29.6	7.3	189	14.5	2.6
Ham, boiled, lean and fat	16.3	39.6	435	12.7	2.5
Kidney, sheeps', fried	28.0	9.1	199	16.6	14.5
Liver, calves, fried	29.0	14.5	262	8.8	21.7
Luncheon meat, canned	11.4	29.0	335	17.5	1.1
Pork, leg, roast	24.6	23.2	317	5.2	1.7
Sausage, pork, fried	11.5	24.8	326	19.7	3.3
Sausage, beef, fried	13.8	18.4	287	21.2	4.1
Mutton, leg, roast	25.0	20.4	292	4.3	4.3

FISH

Fish can be divided into two categories according to the area of the sea they inhabit.

Pelagic fish live in the middle and surface layers of the sea, examples are herrings, mackerel, pilchards and sprats. These fish feed on algae and plankton and generally have a high fat content, ie 20%.

Demersal fish inhabit the bottom of the sea, examples are cod, plaice, sole and haddock. These fish feed on plankton, worms and molluscs. Their fat content is 0.5-5%.

Fish are further classified according to the percentage of fat in their flesh.
1   *Low fat group* with less than 5% fat. There are three subdivisions in this group.
(a)   Fish with high protein content, eg cod and haddock.
(b)   Fish with a very high protein content, eg tuna and halibut.

Nutritional Value of Fish

(c) Fish with a low protein content, eg shellfish.
2 *Medium fat group* containing 5-15% fat, eg salmon and kippers.
3 *High fat group* containing over 15% fat, eg herrings, sardines and sprats.

During the last 20 years many new fishing regions have been developed. The annual world catch of fish is 61 million tonnes. Marine fishing is declining in spite of increased efforts to increase the catch. In the 1950s whales provided up to 10% of the world's marine catch, now the catch has declined to only 2% of the total catch, representing 1 million tonnes per year. A large proportion of the fish caught are used to provide fishmeal for animal food.

Fish flesh consists of muscle fibres which contain colloidal protein. On cooking the protein coagulates and the flesh becomes opaque. A few extractives are formed. Overcooking results in shrinkage, toughening of the muscle and a loss of water and extractives.

Fish must be eaten as fresh as possible. It is a highly perishable food and for this reason a high percentage of fish is preserved by freezing it. Fish usually struggle in the fishing nets before they die resulting in a depletion of glycogen and therefore no lactic acid is formed which would act as a preservative in the dead fish.

The consumption of fish in the UK per head per year is about 16.6 lb (7.54 kg); which considering we are surrounded by sea is a low intake.

Nutritional value of fish
Protein
   Fish contains a little less protein than meat as it has a higher percentage of water. The protein is of high biological value.
Fat
   The fat content of fish varies from less than 1% to 25% according to the type of fish eaten.
Carbohydrate
   Very little carbohydrate is present in fish.
Minerals
   Fish is a good source of iodine, phosphorus, fluorine and calcium. The intake of calcium from canned fish such as sardines is high as the soft bones are eaten. Fish generally is not a good source of iron.
Vitamins
   Vitamin A is found in fatty fish, eg herrings, salmon and sardines. There is no vitamin A in white fish such as cod, haddock and plaice.
Vitamin B complex
   Fish contains the vitamins of the B complex in similar quantities to those found in meat.
Vitamin C
   Only a trace present.
Vitamin D
   Vitamin D is found in fatty fish and not in white fish. Cod and halibut liver oils are exceptionally rich sources of vitamins A and D.

Meat, Poultry and Fish

Nutritional value of fish per 100 g

Fish	Protein g	Fat g	Calories	Calcium mg	Iron mg
Cod, fried	20.7	4.7	140	49.6	1.0
Haddock, steamed	22.0	0.8	97	54.6	0.7
Herring, fried	21.8	15.1	235	38.6	1.9
Kippers, baked	23.2	11.4	201	64.8	1.4
Mackerel, fried	20.0	11.3	187	28.4	1.2
Plaice, fried	18.0	14.4	234	44.9	0.8
Prawns	21.2	1.8	104	145.0	1.1
Salmon, canned	19.7	6.0	137	66.4	1.3
Sardines, canned	20.4	22.6	294	409.0	4.0
Trout, steamed	22.3	4.5	133	35.8	1.0

PRACTICAL WORK ON MEAT AND FISH

EXPERIMENT 1

Experiment to determine the percentage moisture in a sample of meat

Place 5 g of finely ground meat sample into a weighed evaporating dish. Dry in an oven slowly until constant weight is reached.

$$\% \text{ moisture} = \frac{\text{Initial weight of meat} - \text{Final weight} \times 100\%}{\text{Initial weight}}$$

	% water
Beef steak, raw	68.3
Chicken, roast	61.1
Liver, raw	71.6
Mutton chop, raw, lean and fat	32.3
Pork, raw, lean only	74.9
Pork sausage, fried	48.5

EXPERIMENT 2

Examination of meat and fish under the microscope

Place a scraping of meat on a microscope slide and stain it with Ehrlich's Haemotoxylin, examine the muscle fibres under the microscope. Repeat with a sample of fish.

Practical Work

EXPERIMENT 3

Examination of raw and cooked meat
Obtain samples of beef, lamb and pork. Examine the samples noting distribution of fat and connective tissue and the colour, pH and smell of each sample. Boil each sample in water and examine the cooked products. Note the temperature at which coagulation of the proteins occurs.

EXPERIMENT 4

Experiment to determine the cooking losses which occur when meat is cooked
Take 200 g of rump steak, 1 pork chop, 1 lamb chop and 200 g of liver. Weigh each sample and place each sample on a piece of aluminium foil. Grill each sample and weigh the meat and the extractives formed in each case. Calculate the percentage loss in weight for each sample.

% loss of weight on cooking =

$$\frac{\text{Weight of raw meat} - \text{Weight of cooked meat} \times 100\%}{\text{Weight of raw meat}}$$

This experiment can be repeated for a sample of fish and a chicken joint.

EXPERIMENT 5

Experiment to show the effects of cooking a meat sample in a microwave oven
Take two samples of grilling steak and weigh them. Cook one sample in a microwave oven and the other sample by grilling until well done. Weigh each sample when cooked. Compare cooking losses, quantity of extractives formed, colour, flavour and texture of each sample.

EXPERIMENT 6

To test meat for the presence of protein
Place some scrapings from a piece of meat in a test tube and add some Millon's reagent. A red colour, formed on heating, indicates the presence of protein. Repeat with fish, chicken and sausage.

EXPERIMENT 7

To determine the presence of starch in sausages
Boil a small piece of sausage for 10 minutes. Place the sample on a

Meat, Poultry and Fish

slide and add iodine solution; a blue-black colour indicates the presence of starch. Starch containing substances such as breadcrumbs are used as fillers in sausages.

11
Cereals

Cereals form an important part of the diet in most communities of the world. In parts of Asia and Africa cereals can provide 90% of the total Calorie intake. In Great Britain cereals provide about 25% of our Calories.

Cereals are the seeds of the domestic grasses; the principal ones being rice, wheat, maize, barley, oats, rye and millets.

Nutritive values of common cereals

Per 100 g	Calories	Protein g	Fat g	Water g	Calcium mg	Iron mg	B1 mg	B2 mg	Nicotinic acid mg
Wheat	334	12.2	2.3	13.7	30	3.5	0.40	0.17	5.0
Rice (husked)	357	7.5	1.0	9.6	15	2.8	0.25	0.12	4.0
Maize	356	9.5	4.3	10.9	12	5.0	0.33	0.13	1.5
Barley	350	10.5	2.2	12.0	35	4.0	0.50	0.20	7.0
Oats	385	13.0	7.5	12.9	60	3.8	0.50	0.14	1.3
Rye	319	11.0	1.9	13.8	50	3.5	0.27	0.10	1.2
Millets	343	10.1	3.3	11.1	30	6.2	0.40	0.12	3.5

RICE

Rice forms the staple food of more than half the world's population. It contains less protein than the other common cereals but the protein is of high quality. Most rice is grown in water, but some is grown on dry land. When the crop is ripe it is cut and threshed. It is then milled to remove the outer husk and then milled again to remove the brown bran surrounding the grain. Pearling the rice produces a white grain known as polished rice which can be treated further to produce a greater sheen.

Cereals

A high proportion of the thiamine content of the rice is found in the outside layers of the grain thus the dehusking and polishing process considerably reduce the nutritional value of rice in this respect. When rice is dehusked it contains 4.0 microgrammes of thiamine and by the time it has been polished twice it contains only 1.0 microgramme of thiamine per gramme of rice.

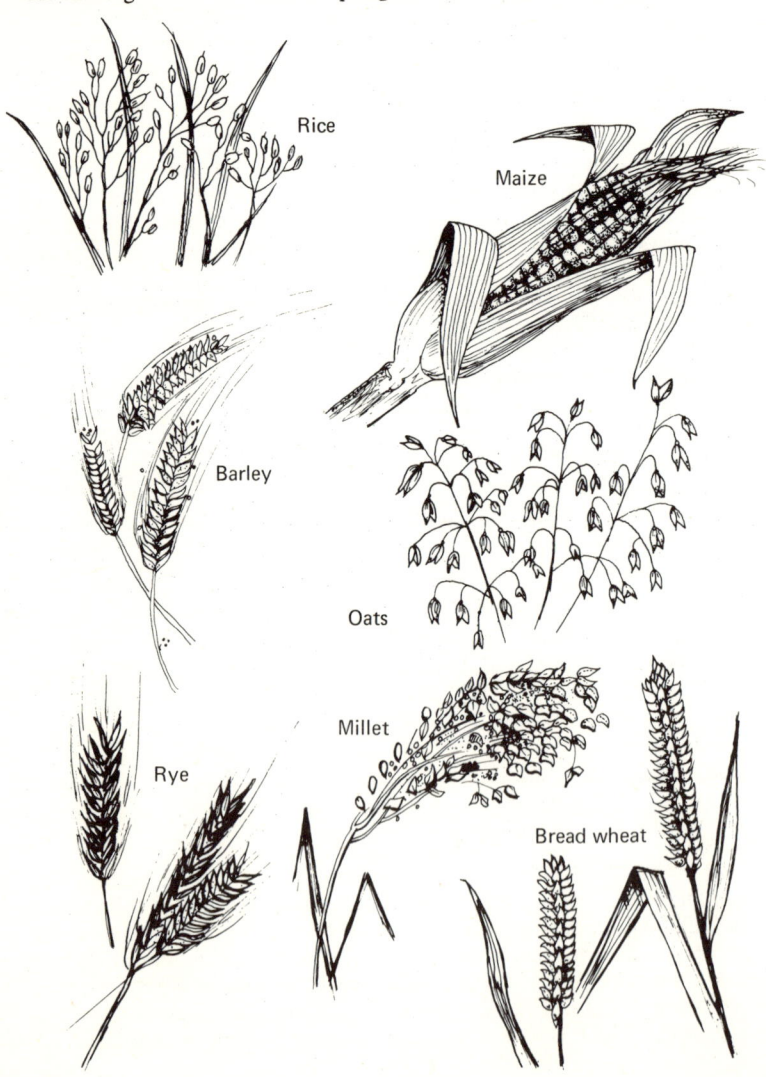

Rice

Maize

Barley

Oats

Rye

Millet

Bread wheat

Experimental cooking of rice

Rice contains a pigment called *flavone* which is white in an acid medium and yellow in an alkaline medium.

Method

1 Boil ½ litre of salted tap water. Add 28 g of rice and cook until soft.
2 Boil ½ litre of salted tap water containing 1 teaspoonful of lemon juice. Add 28 g of rice and cook until soft.
3 Boil ½ litre of salted tap water containing 1 teaspoonful of bicarbonate of soda. Add 28 g of rice and cook until soft.

Take the pH of the cooking water in each case. Note colour of the cooked rice and comment on the pH of tap water and its effect on the flavone.

MAIZE

This cereal is widely used in South America, South and East Africa as a human food. In this country we use it as the vegetable corn-on-the-cob and in cornflakes and cornflour. It does not contain gluten so it cannot be used for bread. Nicotinic acid is present as the compound niacytin which cannot be absorbed by the body.

In Latin America the maize is ground and cooked into cakes called tortillas. Before the maize is ground the Latin Americans soak the maize in lime water, this softens the grains and also has the effect of releasing the nicotinic acid from the niacytin. Thus the Latin Americans are able to keep free of the nicotinic acid deficiency disease pellagra.

In Africa the maize is boiled into a porridge.

Maize contains poor quality protein compared with other cereals. The yellow maize is a good source of carotene, the precursor of vitamin A. Maize or corn oil is a very important cooking oil.

BARLEY

Most barley grown in the British Isles is used for beer and whisky manufacture. For beer making the barley grains are allowed to germinate and then they are dried and the malt is then used for brewing. The malt contains amylases which convert starch into sugars which can then be fermented by yeasts into alcohol and carbon dioxide.

If the husk of the barley is removed and the grain is ground, pearl barley is formed which is used in soups and stews.

OATS

This cereal is mainly grown for animal food, but some is used for making porridge oats and oatcakes.

RYE

This is the only cereal other than wheat which contains enough gluten for breadmaking. It forms the main bread grain in Scandinavia

Cereals

and East European countries. Rye bread has a poor crumb compared with wheat bread. Rye is used to make rye crispbread.

PRACTICAL WORK

Obtain a sample of rye flour and use it in a bread recipe. Compare texture, crust, flavour and colour with bread made from wheat flour.

MILLETS

Millets are used as cereals in Asia and Africa. Their nutritional value is good. They are usually made into porridge or ground into a meal.

WHEAT

Wheat is mainly grown in Canada, Australia, Argentine, India, Russia, China and Great Britain. The wheat from the various countries have different characteristics and have to be blended together to obtain the best quality flour. About 356 millions tonnes of wheat are produced annually in the world and it is eaten by approximately half the world's population.

The wheat berry

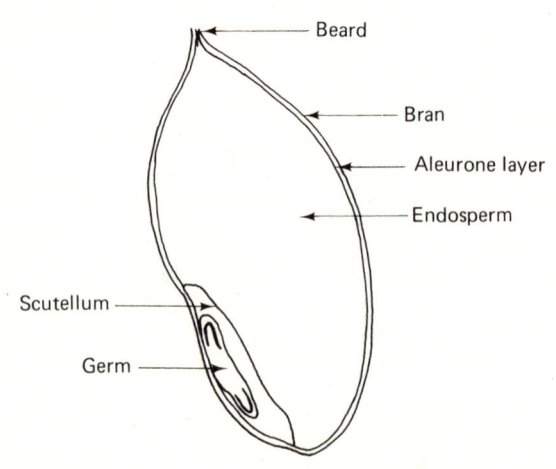

Practical Work

Approximate composition of the wheat berry

	% by weight		% by weight
Carbohydrate	66-73		
Water	14	Endosperm	85
Protein	7-14	Bran	13
Fat	1.0	Germ	2
Minerals	0.6		

A wheat grain is 6 mm long and about 3 mm wide. It has a crease running along its length. At one end it has some hairy tufts called the beard. The outside layer is called the bran. Under the bran there are several layers, the inner one being the aleurone layer which is rich in protein. The central part of the grain consists of the floury endosperm which makes up 80-90% of the grain. The germ is found at the base of the grain and this is the embryo plant which is rich in fats, proteins, B vitamins, vitamin E and iron.

Strong and weak wheats

Wheats vary in composition according to their variety, the climate, the fertility of the soil, etc. They are classified by their protein content. Canadian wheat is classified as a strong wheat, this means that it has a high protein content and the flour milled from it will produce a loaf with a good volume. This type of flour is also useful for rich pastries and batters.

The most important protein in wheat is called gluten, this protein has the ability to form strong elastic threads when it absorbs water.

Most wheats grown in Great Britain have a low protein content and are called weak wheats. Weak flour produces products with less rise than strong flour and the texture is softer. Weak flour is used for cake and biscuit making.

Hardness and softness of wheat are milling characteristics referring to the way the grains break down when they are milled.

The milling of wheat

Wheat was first milled with stones in hand mills and later in wind and water mills. Over 100 years ago the steel roller mill was developed and this is the machine that is used today. This process separates the endosperm from the bran producing fine white flour.

An outline of the milling process

1   Wheat is transported to storage silos.
2   Wheat is cleaned by sifting out foreign bodies and washing.
3   The wheat is dried to an agreed moisture content. If the wheat is

too dry it will be too brittle for milling. If the wheat is too moist it clogs the rollers.
4   Wheat is taken to the first break rollers which are grooved steel rollers rotating at different speeds. The rollers break the grain and scrape some of the endosperm from the bran. The broken wheat is sieved and some flour is formed at this stage. The middle sized particles of bran and endosperm are known as middlings or semolina.
5   The middlings travel to the purifier which separates out more flour from the bran by a system of sieves.
6   The coarse particles of bran from the first break rollers travel to the second break rollers where they are broken down into smaller particles. Some more flour is formed from the second break rollers and this is sieved off from the middlings which go to the middlings purifier and the large particles go to the third break rollers.
7   This process continues until after the fifth break rollers the large particles of bran are mainly free of endosperm. The bran particles are used for animal feeding or for breakfast cereals.
8   The flour formed from each stage is blended. The miller usually blends flour from strong and weak wheats to give a flour with desirable baking qualities.
    Wheatgerm does not appear in ordinary white flour as it is rich in fat which tends to go rancid and spoil the colour and flavour of the flour.

The bleaching of flour
As the customer demands really white flour, the flour is bleached using a chemical bleaching agent. Dyox, chlorine dioxide is widely used in Britain, USA and Canada as a bleaching agent.

Improving flour
As flour matures its baking qualities improve. Matured flour produces loaves of larger volume and a finer textured crumb than immature flour.
Improving or maturing agents can be added to the flour. These agents do not increase carbon dioxide production in the fermented dough but they improve gas retention as the dough is made more elastic.
Chlorine dioxide is a common improving agent as well as being a bleaching agent. Vitamin C can also be used as an improver. It speeds up the development of the gluten strands in the dough and cuts down the rising time.
Self raising flour is made from weak wheat which has sodium bicarbonate and acid calcium phosphate added to it as raising agents.

Extraction rates of flour
If flour is wholewheat then it is 100% extraction and contains all the original bran that surrounds the wheat, the endosperm and the germ.

When white flour is made the coarse bran particles and the wheat germ are removed. Most white flour consumed in this country is 70% extraction; ie 30% of the original wheat grain, mainly the bran, does not appear in the flour. 70% extraction flour has a good colour and favourable baking qualities. Unfortunately when this flour is made parts of the grain not included contain vitamins of the B complex, calcium and iron. The loss of these valuable nutrients is not ignored as nutritional supplements are added by law to all white flours.

All flours must contain not less than
    0.24 mg of vitamin B1
    1.65 mg of iron   per 100 g of flour

Calcium is added to flours, except for some self raising and wholemeal flour so that the calcium content of the flour is not less than 235 mg and not more than 390 mg in 100 g of flour.

Flour is primarily used in this country to make bread. Flour has an important part to play in the nutrition of the population. There seems to be no appreciable difference between the nutritional value of white and brown flours. Wholemeal breads contain more roughage than white bread.

Percentage of intake of nutrients provided by bread per person per day

Protein	17.0	
Energy value	14.4	
Carbohydrate	25.5	
Calcium	13.4	
Iron	17.7	Figures from *Household Food*
Thiamine	22.1	*Consumption and Expenditure 1972*

The composition of bread per 100 g

	Water	Protein	Fat	Carbo-hydrate	Cals	Calcium	Iron	B1	B2	Nicotinic acid
	g	g	g	g		mg	mg	mg	mg	mg
White	38.4	8.0	1.4	51.7	240	91	1.82	0.18	-	1.7
Energen Rolls	8.5	44.0	4.1	45.7	390	46	3.96	0.18	-	1.7
Milk bread	34.5	10.7	2.4	50.3	255	140	1.77	0.19	0.08	1.7
Brown bread	37.7	8.7	2.1	49.9	242	95	2.44	0.21	-	2.5
Wholemeal	40.1	8.2	2.0	47.1	228	26	2.88	0.20	0.10	3.5
Hovis	39.7	9.0	2.3	47.6	237	107	2.68	0.29	-	2.0

Cereals

Brown bread must contain not less than 0.6% fibre and can be coloured using caramel.
Wholemeal bread is made from the whole grain including the germ. No bleach or improver can be added.
Wheatgerm breads eg Hovis. The germ is cooked to destroy the enzymes which would speed up rancidity. The germ is then blended with flour which contains some bran.

Wheat is used in the production of breakfast cereals and pasta such as spaghetti, macaroni and lasagne. Hard Durum wheats are used for making pasta.

Nutritional value of pasta per 100 g

Calories	380
Carbohydrates	75g
Protein	12g
Vit B1	0.09 mg
Vit B2	0.1 mg
Calcium	10 mg
Iron	1.2 mg
Phosphorus	144 mg

Baking technology

When a dough is made strong gluten threads develop. Yeast ferments sugars to form the raising agent, carbon dioxide. The heat of the oven coagulates the protein and partially gelatinises the starch granules.

When water is added to the bread flour gluten strands are formed. Enzymes (amylases) present in the flour start to break down the starch into maltose. Only the damaged starch granules are attacked by the amylases at this stage. Yeast cannot act on the starch so these enzymes are of great importance.

The flour contains about 2% sugar and this provides an immediate substrate for the yeast. The maltose is split into glucose by the enzyme maltase which is present in the yeast. Any sucrose present is split into fructose and glucose by sucrase which is also found in yeast. The yeast then uses the glucose and fructose to form carbon dioxide and alcohol.

$$C_6H_{12}O_6 \xrightarrow[\text{in yeast}]{\text{zymases}} 2C_2H_5OH + 2CO_2$$

glucose ←ethanol

The carbon dioxide is held in the gluten network and the dough is left to rise. When the dough has approximately doubled its size it is kneaded again to redistribute the ingredients so that the yeast has some sugar surrounding it. The dough is left to rise further and then it is cooked. When the dough is in the oven, starch granules are disrupted by heat and more starch is broken down to maltose by amylases. The maltose can then be broken down to glucose while the heat penetration is not great enough to break down the enzymes. The oven temperature stops the yeast fermentation but the carbon dioxide expands, the proteins coagulate and the starch partially gelatinises. If there is inadequate amylase in the flour the bread will be under fermented and the crust pale.

BREADMAKING   EXPERIMENT 1
Standard recipe

        100 g of bread flour   5 g of yeast
        1.5 g of salt   65 ml of water

Method
1   Weigh flour into 20 cm basin and make two wells in it.
2   Measure 65 ml of water in a measuring cylinder and warm to 25°C.
3   Dissolve 1.5 g of salt in half the water in a small bowl.
4   Mix 5 g of yeast with half the water in a small bowl.
5   Add liquid from each bowl to the 2 wells in the flour. Note the time.
6   Mix dough for 1 minute using 60 strokes.
7   Place the dough in a glass beaker, mark the level of the dough with a glass marker. Place beaker in a prover which should be at 25°C. Note time taken for it to double in size.
8   Remove the dough from the prover and knock back using 40 strokes.
9   Place the dough in a greased bread tin and put in the prover until it has doubled in size.
10   Bake in the oven for 20 minutes at 475°F.

EXPERIMENT 2

Experiment to show the effect of varying the ingredients in breadmaking
Prepare 1 loaf using the standard recipe and then 1 loaf using each of the following variations to the recipe but using the standard method.
1   Use cake flour instead of bread flour.
2   Use 2 g of yeast.
3   Use 10 g of yeast.
4   Use 45 ml of water.
5   Use 90 ml of water.
6   Omit the salt.
7   Use 5 g of salt.
8   Use 15 g of salt.
9   Add 20 g of sugar to the yeast and water mixture.
10   Add 10 g of lard to the flour.

Results
    Examine all the loaves for texture, colour, size and flavour.

Cereals

Loaf 1 It is not possible to develop strong gluten threads in cake flour thus there is no firm framework for the carbon dioxide to be held in. The loaf is small with a close, uneven texture.

Loaf 2 The 2 g of yeast present is inadequate for the amount of flour used. When this yeast ferments there is insufficient carbon dioxide produced to raise the dough. The loaf is therefore smaller than the standard and has a poor flavour.

Loaf 3 The excess amount of yeast produces a loaf that has risen excessively. The texture is coarse as large bubbles of carbon dioxide were produced. The yeast flavour of the loaf is too strong.

Loaf 4 There is insufficient water for the formation of elastic gluten threads. The dough is strong and inelastic. The loaf is small as the threads are too strong for the usual leavening reaction to take place.

Loaf 5 The dough is very wet and too elastic. The resulting loaf is small and has a coarse texture.

Loaf 6 The loaf is slightly larger than the standard as the salt inhibits yeast fermentation. Texture is a little coarse and the flavour is poor. The loaf will probably stale quickly as the salt would normally hold the moisture.

Loaf 7 Salt is a powerful inhibitor of fermentation. Salt also makes the gluten more stable and less extensible. The loaf is smaller than the standard, it is hard with a poor texture, colour and flavour.

Loaf 8 Same effect as 7 only more marked.

Loaf 9 Sugar increases the gas production so the loaf is larger. The yeast is unable to ferment all the sugar and a browning reaction takes place on the crust of the loaf giving it a characteristic foxy-red colour.

Loaf 10 The lard gives the loaf an improved flavour, increased volume and a softer, moister texture. The bread will also have improved keeping qualities.

Conclusion

It is necessary to add the ingredients in exactly the right proportions in order to obtain a loaf of the correct volume which has a good texture, colour and flavour.

EXPERIMENT 3

Experiment to show the effect of ascorbic acid (vitamin C) on a bread dough

Recipe

100 g of bread flour 65 ml of water
1.5 g of salt 5 mg of ascorbic acid
5 g of yeast

Method

The same as experiment (1) for 1, 2, 3, 4, 5 and 6, but dissolve the ascorbic acid in the water with the salt.

Practical Work

7 Place the dough formed in (6) in a greased bread tin. Leave in the prover to double its size.
8 Bake in the oven for 20 mins at 475°F.

Results
A good quality loaf is produced with good flavour, texture and volume.

Conclusion
Ascorbic acid effectively cuts down the proving time. Its effect on the dough is to speed up the development of the gluten threads.

EXPERIMENT 4

Experiment to show the effect of salt on gluten
Method
Form three gluten balls by kneading together bread flour and water. Attach a thread to each. Place the first ball in a bowl containing water so that the ball does not touch the sides or the bottom of the bowl; this can be done by tying the thread to a rod placed across the top of the bowl. Place the second ball in a bowl containing a salt solution of medium concentration and the third ball in a bowl containing a strong salt solution. Observe the gluten balls noting any changes which occur.

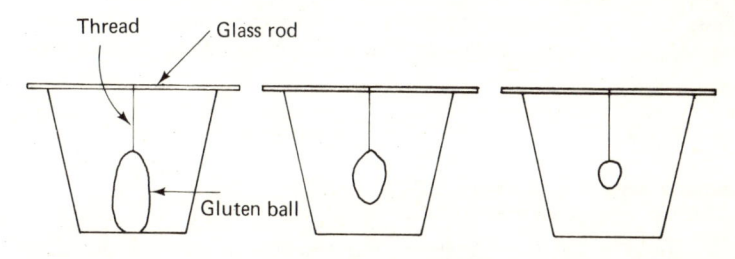

Thread   Glass rod
Gluten ball

Gluten ball in water. Gluten expands and becomes very elastic.

Gluten ball in medium concentration salt solution. Gluten shrinks and becomes tougher.

Gluten ball in strong salt solution. Gluten shrinks and becomes very tough.

Conclusion
Salt makes gluten less extensible and tougher.

EXPERIMENT 5

Experiment to show that weak cake flour contains less gluten than strong bread flour
Method
Mix 50 g of cake flour with sufficient water to moisten all the flour.

Cereals

Work into a dough. Stretch dough with the hands and note its elasticity. Repeat using strong bread flour.
Results
Cake flour forms very weak gluten strands, while the bread flour forms a strong dough with elastic threads.
Conclusion
Cake flour does not contain enough gluten to form a strong extensible dough and is therefore unsuitable for breadmaking.

Raising agents

1 Biological
Yeast is an example of a biological raising agent; its action is described in the section on bread making.

2 Chemical
The action of an acid on sodium bicarbonate produces carbon dioxide which is used as a leavening agent in many baked products. Sodium bicarbonate produces carbon dioxide when heated but a residue of sodium carbonate remains which has an undesirable alkaline taste.
There are several acids which can be combined with sodium bicarbonate to form baking powder. Cream of tartar (potassium hydrogen tartrate) is commonly used but acid calcium phosphate is also used.

$$\begin{array}{c} \text{CHOHCOOH} \\ | \\ \text{CHOHCOOK} \end{array} + \text{NaHCO}_3 \xrightarrow{\text{heat}} \begin{array}{c} \text{CHOHCOONa} \\ | \\ \text{CHOHCOOK} \end{array} + CO_2 + H_2O$$

potassium hydrogen tartrate   sodium bicarbonate   sodium potassium tartrate

Cream of tartar is preferable to tartaric acid in a baking powder as less carbon dioxide is evolved when it comes into contact with moisture but in the heat of the oven a large volume of carbon dioxide is evolved.
Commercial baking powders contain a diluent which separates the acid and the sodium bicarbonate and helps to keep the product dry.

EXPERIMENTS

Experiment 1
Place a small amount of sodium bicarbonate in each of two test tubes. Heat one with water and the second tube heat dry. Test gas evolved from each tube with lime water and taste the residues.

Practical Work

Experiment 2
Place a small quantity of sodium bicarbonate in a test tube and heat dry until no more carbon dioxide is evolved. Cool, add a few drops of dilute hydrochloric acid. Test for carbon dioxide. Acid causes more carbon dioxide to be evolved.

Experiment 3
Place 1 teaspoonful of sodium bicarbonate in a test tube with 2 teaspoonsful of cream of tartar. Half fill the test tube with water. Heat, test gas evolved with lime water. Taste the residue and compare with residues formed in experiment (1).

Experiment 4

Experiment to compare raising agents used for scones
Basic recipe
    114 g of plain flour   Pinch of salt
    1½ level teaspoonsful of raising agent   21 g of fat
                                         70 ml of milk

Make scones in the normal way and roll out to 12 mm thickness. Use the following mixtures as raising agents.

1. ½ level teaspoonful of sodium bicarbonate and 1 level teaspoonful of cream of tartar.
2. 1½ level teaspoonsful of sodium bicarbonate.
3. 1½ level teaspoonsful of commercial baking powder.
4. 1½ level teaspoonsful of cream of tartar.
5. ½ level teaspoonful of sodium bicarbonate.
6. 1 level teaspoonful of cream of tartar.
7. No raising agent.

Measure the height of the scones produced and examine them for colour, texture and flavour. Which raising agent is the most suitable for scones?

12
Starches

Plants are able to convert sugars formed in photosynthesis into a more complex chemical called starch. Starch is stored in plants in roots, eg in the parsnip, turnip and swede, in tubers, eg in the potato and yams, in underground stems, eg arrowroot, and in the fruit, eg in the apple, banana and in cereals.

Starch forms the basis of the diet of many millions of human beings and animals. It is regularly consumed in rice, maize, wheat, rye, yams, cassava, barley and potatoes.

Starch is formed as granules in small bodies called leucoplasts. The appearance and properties of the starch granules are characteristic for each plant. Starches are not readily available for digestion in raw foods as they are covered by a cellulose cell wall. When the food is cooked this wall is softened and starch is then available.

The extraction of starch from wheat
Soak wheat grains in water overnight. Peel off the bran. Add water to the wheat and grind with a pestle and mortar. The oil content of the germ rises to the top as it is less dense than water and is then skimmed off. The protein is suspended in the water and if this is removed the starch is left at the bottom of the vessel. Wash and dry the starch. Starch can also be extracted from roots and tubers using this method.

Starch is extracted commercially from cereals, potatoes, cassava and the sweet potato.

Chemical structure of starch
Starch is basically formed from chains of glucose linked together to form very complex molecules. Starch can be separated into two distinct compounds: amylose and amylopectin.

Amylose is the simplest compound consisting of glucose units linked together in a straight chain. Amylose reacts with iodine producing a blue-black colour.

Starches

Amylopectin is more complex consisting of glucose units in short chains which have bridges or connections between them. Amylopectin gives a red or brown colour with iodine solution.

Diagrammatic representation of the structure of amylopectin

The separation of starch into amylose and amylopectin

Take a sample of starch and heat it in water at 65°C. The granules of starch swell and amylose, which is much more soluble in water than amylopectin, dissolves into the water. Amylopectin is left within the starch granules which can be centrifuged off.

Gelatinisation of starch

All starches are insoluble in cold water but when they are heated with water the starch granules suddenly swell taking up water and there is an increase in viscosity. This uptake of water occurs at about 65°C depending on the type of starch used and is called gelatinisation. The uptake of water continues for about 20°; a gel is formed, its clarity and strength depending on the type of starch that is used.

Gelatinisation occurs more readily if the starch granules are damaged as the entry of water into the granules is facilitated. If the granules are crowded hard lumps are formed so starch should be dispersed mechanically while it is heated.

Use of starch in the diet

Starch is used in the diet as a source of energy. When completely oxidised by the cells it provides 4.2 Calories/g.

% Starch content of some common foods

Wheat	64	Arrowroot	25
Potato	20	Maize	68
Tapioca	21.6	Rice	75

Starches

Uses of starch in cookery
The uses of starch in cookery depend on the ability of starch to take up water and gelatinise.
1   Starch grains can be used to make puddings, eg rice pudding, tapioca and semolina.
2   Used in the form of flour in bread, cakes, biscuits, puddings and pastry, etc. Usually only partial gelatinisation takes place in these products as there is insufficient liquid present.
3   It is used to thicken soups, stews and gravy.
4   To make sauces, eg the roux foundation sauce.
5   To make fillings, eg lemon meringue pie filling.
6   To bind and coat fish cakes, croquettes, etc.

EXPERIMENTAL STUDY OF STARCHES

1 The observation of starch granules in the potato
Cut a very thin slice of potato, place on a microscope slide, add a few drops of iodine and cover with a coverslip. Observe the starch granules under the microscope, they should be stained blue-black.

Cook a potato and remove a thin slice from the inside and outside of the potato, stain with iodine and observe under the microscope. What happens to the starch granules when they are cooked? Does the potato cook first on the inside or the outside?

2 Comparison of the appearance of starch granules from different sources
Obtain as many samples of starch as possible, eg wheat flour, cornflour, rice flour, potato starch, arrowroot. Place a little of the starch on a slide and add a few drops of iodine solution, place a coverslip over the top, observe the shape of the granules under the microscope and draw.

3 Experiment to show the effect of heating various suspensions of starch
Take 3 g of various starches and mix each with 50 ml of water. Heat in a water bath starting from cold. Remove 1 drop of each mixture at once and then remove 1 drop at 20°, 40°, 60°, 70°, 80°, 90° and 100°C. Boil each tube for 2 minutes and remove 1 drop from each. Place each drop on a microscope slide, stain with iodine solution and view under the microscope, note swelling of starch granules. Note appearance of the gel formed from each starch and its viscosity. What is the gelatinisation temperature of each starch used?

Potato starch and arrowroot form the clearest gels and thus are used for glazes. After boiling for 2 minutes all starch granules will have burst and a smooth gel is formed.

4 Experiment to show the effect of varying the concentration of starch when preparing a starch gel
Take 6 small beakers, place in them 10, 20, 30, 40, 50 and 60 g of starch respectively. Mix each with 250 ml of water. Heat each one

stirring continuously for the same length of time. Compare the texture, colour, etc of each. Which concentration would be most suitable for (a) a roux foundation sauce and (b) a lemon pie filling?

5 Experiment to show the effects of sugar and acid on a starch gel
Take 6 small beakers and use as follows:
To beaker 1 add 3 g of starch, 50 ml of water and 50 g of sugar
To beaker 2 add 3 g of starch, 50 ml of water and 30 g of sugar
To beaker 3 add 3 g of starch, 50 ml of water and 10 g of sugar
To beaker 4 add 3 g of starch, no water and 50 ml of lemon juice
To beaker 5 add 3 g of starch, 25 ml of water and 25 ml of lemon juice
To beaker 6 add 3 g of starch, 40 ml of water and 10 ml of lemon juice

Heat all 6 beakers in a water bath at 95°C. Observe differences in the viscosity and clarity of the gels formed. Carry out an iodine test on a small sample of the gel from each beaker.
Sugar reduces the strength of the gel as it competes with the starch for water. The starch granules do not have sufficient water for complete gelatinisation. Lemon juice causes the hydrolysis of starch to sugars, thus at high acid concentrations the iodine test may be negative as there is no starch left to give a reaction.

$$\text{Starch} \xrightarrow{\text{Iodine solution}} \text{Blue-black colour}$$

$$\text{Sugars} \xrightarrow{\text{Iodine solution}} \text{Red-brown colour}$$

6 Experiment to illustrate the correct method for the preparation of the roux foundation sauce.
Method
(a)   Take 28 g of margarine and melt it in a pan, add 28 g of flour. Stir continuously and add 280 ml of water gradually.
(b)   Take 28 g of margarine and melt in a pan, add 28 g of flour and then add 280 ml of water quickly with very little stirring.
(c)   Place 28 g of flour in a pan and add 280 ml of warm water gradually and stir continuously.
Results
(a)   A smooth sauce is formed as the fat disperses the starch granules and prevents them from sticking together and forming lumps.
(b)   The sauce formed is lumpy as there is inadequate stirring.
(c)   The sauce formed will again be lumpy as there is no fat to disperse the granules.

13
Sugars

ALL sugars are carbohydrates. They can be classified as monosaccharides or disaccharides.

Monosaccharides
These are chemically made up from one saccharide unit.
Glucose
Glucose is the sugar found in the blood and is present in some fruits and vegetables.
Fructose
Fructose is a very sweet sugar found in ripe fruits and vegetables.
Galactose
Galactose is found in milk as part of the lactose molecule.

Disaccharides
Maltose
Maltose is the breakdown product of starch. When starch is acted upon by amylase in the saliva, maltose is formed.
Lactose
Lactose is only found in mammalian milk. It is mildly sweet.
Sucrose
Sucrose is the most important sugar and is manufactured in green plants in a process called photosynthesis.

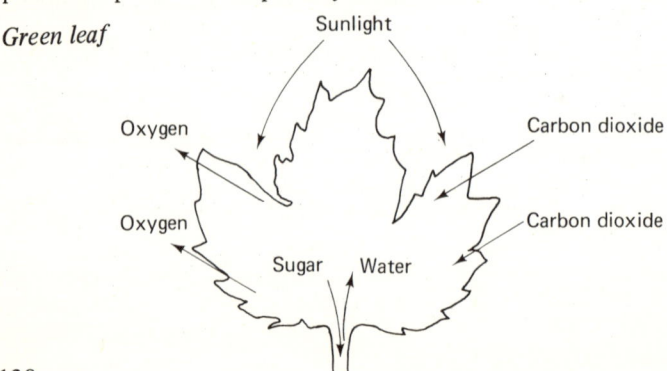

Green leaf

Sugars

This reaction which takes place in bodies called chloroplasts can be shown in a simplified form in the equation:

Carbon dioxide + Water + Energy from sunlight $\xrightarrow{\text{Chlorophyll}}$ Sucrose + Oxygen

$$12\ CO_2 + 11\ H_2O + \text{Energy} \xrightarrow{\text{Chlorophyll}} C_{12}H_{22}O_{11} + 12O_2$$

Relative sweetness of sugars

Sucrose	= 1	Lactose	= 0.16
Fructose	= 1.7	Maltose	= 0.32
Glucose	= 0.7	Galactose	= 0.32

Sucrose is found in high concentrations in sugar cane and sugar beet, but all green plants have some sugar in their roots, stems, leaves and fruits.

Sugar cane

Sugar cane provides 60% of the world's supply of sugar and is mainly grown in the tropics. Its appearance is similar to a bamboo and it has a height of 2-6 m. The cane is cut down 12-24 months after planting depending on the local conditions. The cut cane contains 14-17% sucrose.

Sugar beet

Sugar beet was shown to contain sugar by a German chemist in 1747. It is the most important source of sugar in the temperate climates of Europe, USA and Canada. The plant is a biennial and has the ability to store sugar in the root during the first year and then it is lifted. The beet contains 15-20% sucrose. Sugar beet provides 40% of the world's sugar.

Sugar was first mentioned as a food in about 300 BC. This sugar was extracted from sugar cane which was first grown in the South Pacific. In 1264 sugar made its way to England but only the very rich could afford it. Sugar refining began in England in 1554.

Extraction of sugar from the cane

The cane is cut and then taken to the factory where it is shredded, crushed and squeezed. Water is then added to the pulp to extract the juice. Lime is added to the juice and the mixture is heated; lime removes impurities. The juice is then concentrated by evaporation. The resulting juice is then boiled under a vacuum to give a mixture of crystals and syrup. The raw cane sugar crystals are then centrifuged off from the syrup. The syrup is called cane molasses and is used for making rum and industrial alcohol. The raw sugar crystals which are 96% sucrose are transported to a refinery.

Refining of the raw sugar

The raw sugar crystals have an outer coating of molasses and this is removed by mixing the crystals with a warm syrup. The purified crystals are then centrifuged off from the syrup. The crystals are

Sugars

dissolved in water and lime is added. The mixture is treated with carbon dioxide and chalk is formed from the lime. The chalk acts as a trap for impurities. The chalk and impurities are filtered off. The colour is removed by passing the liquid through bone charcoal.

The decolourised liquid is next boiled under a vacuum and some crystals are introduced which bring about crystallisation. The crystals formed are centrifuged off, dried and graded. Large crystals are used to make granulated sugar, and smaller crystals are used for castor sugar. The remaining liquid syrup can be used to form golden syrup or soft brown sugar.

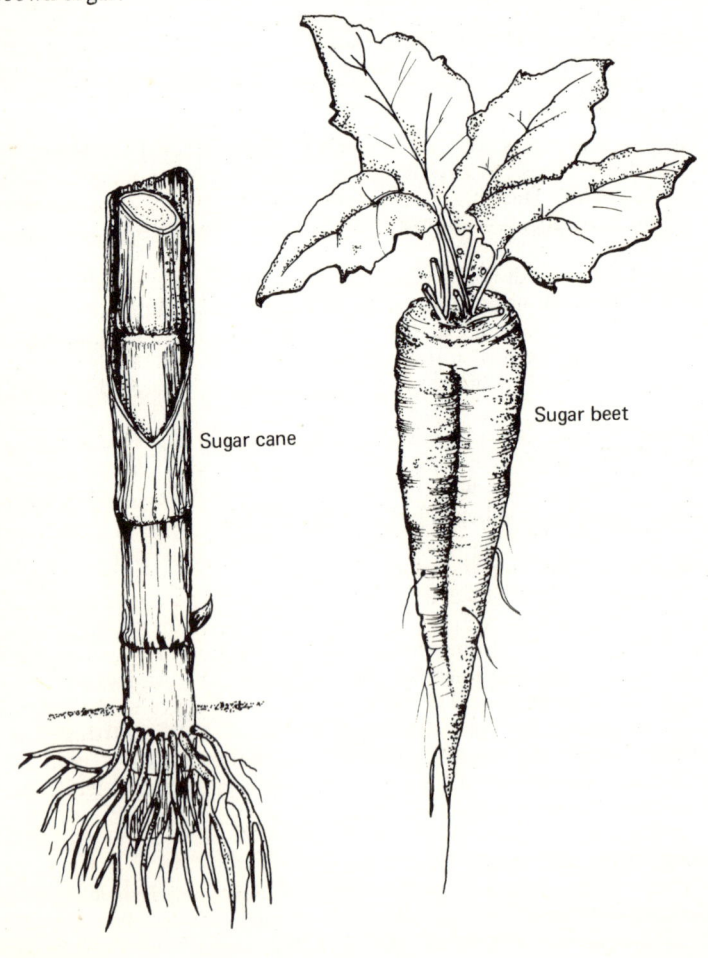

Sugar cane

Sugar beet

Sugars

The refined white sugar crystals are 99.99% pure sucrose. Brown sugars are made from the syrup before it is highly refined and decolourised.

Properties of sucrose
Sucrose is a white crystalline substance with a melting point of 160°C. If heated beyond its melting point it becomes straw coloured, then brown forming caramel at 180°C, dark caramel at 190°C, Black Jack at 210°C and beyond this temperature it decomposes.
Sucrose will give a negative Fehling's test.
It is readily soluble in water. Cold water can dissolve double its own weight of sugar. Sugar raises the boiling point and the density of water.
Sucrose is a concentrated form of energy providing 393 Calories per 100 g.

Uses of sucrose in cookery
1   It is used as a sweetening agent, improving the palatability of many foods.
2   Sugar is a preserving agent in canned and bottled fruits, jams, jellies, sweetened condensed milk and chutneys, etc.
Bacteria present in these products are surrounded by a concentrated sugar solution. By osmosis, water is drawn out of the bacterial cell through their semipermeable cell walls and the bacteria are inactivated as they cannot survive without water.
3   Sugar helps to give a finer taste and texture to canned and bottled fruits. If fruits are surrounded by water, by osmosis water will move from the water into the cells of the fruit, the fruit will swell and the flavour will be diluted. If the syrup surrounding the fruit is too concentrated water will move from the fruit into the surrounding syrup and the fruit will shrink. Thus it is important to ensure that the syrup is the correct concentration so that the bottled fruit will be of a high quality.
4   Sugar is a vital constituent in gel formation in jams, jellies and marmalade. Pectin and acid in fruit together with sugar and water form a gel.

$$\text{Pectin} + \text{Acid} + \text{Sugar} + \text{Water} \xrightarrow{\text{Heat}} \text{A GEL}$$

5   Sugar is used in the preparation of sweets, chocolate and icing.
6   Sugar lightens mixtures as it enables fats to trap air.
7   Sugar stabilises egg white foam and enables the foam to retain a greater proportion of air.
8   Sugar helps to disperse the protein molecules in a flour mixture keeping the gluten soft and increasing the volume of the mixture.
9   Sugar in the form of caramel is used to give flavour and colour to certain products.
10   Sugar acts as a substrate for yeast in fermentation reactions, carbon

Sugars

dioxide and alcohol being the products formed.
11   Sugar gives a brown crust to baked goods.

Sugar boiling

A sugar boiling thermometer

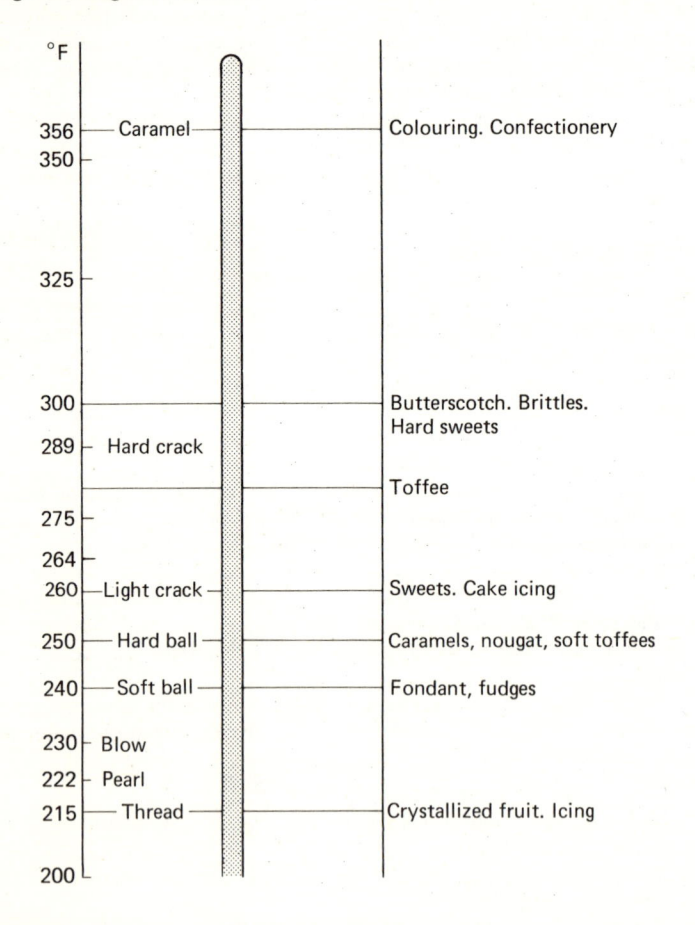

°F		
356	— Caramel —	Colouring. Confectionery
350		
325		
300		Butterscotch. Brittles. Hard sweets
289	— Hard crack	
		Toffee
275		
264		
260	— Light crack —	Sweets. Cake icing
250	— Hard ball —	Caramels, nougat, soft toffees
240	— Soft ball —	Fondant, fudges
230	— Blow	
222	— Pearl	
215	— Thread —	Crystallized fruit. Icing
200		

When sugar is heated it goes through various stages which are utilised in sugar confectionary.
These changes can be studied if 1 kg of sugar is mixed with 250 ml of water and heated gradually in a saucepan. A sugar boiling thermometer must be used.

Sugars

The thread stage   215°F   102°C

If a little of the sugar mixture is extracted when the temperature reaches 215°F and it is placed between the thumb and first finger and the digits are moved apart threads will form.

The pearl stage   222°F   106°C

A thread formed between the fingers at this stage can be stretched. The sugar boils and forms small balls like pearls.

The blow or souffle stage   230°F   110°C

The bubbles in the mixture begin to look like snowflakes at this temperature.

Soft ball stage   240°F   116°C

The syrup begins to thicken at this stage. If a small quantity of the syrup is removed and plunged into cold water it will form a soft ball.

Hard ball stage   250°F   121°C

When a small quantity of syrup is removed and placed in cold water it forms a hard ball.

Light crack stage   264°F   129°C

The syrup begins to turn a pale yellow colour. If a wetted finger is dipped into the surface of the syrup and then plunged into cold water a thin layer of sugar is formed and this falls off the finger. If put in the mouth the sugar sticks to the teeth.

Hard crack stage   289°F   143°C

Dip wetted finger into the syrup and immediately plunge it into cold water, the sugar detaches itself from the finger in thin films and cracks like glass.

Caramel stage   356°F   180°C

The syrup contains very little water at this stage, it becomes darker in colour and it loses its sweetness.

Experiment to show that yeast ferments sugar

Apparatus
As shown in the diagram

Reagents
Yeast, sugar and lime water

Method
Prepare a sugar solution and place it in the flask. Add some yeast to the solution, fresh or dried yeast can be used. Heat flask gently to 40°C. Any gas evolved will pass through the delivery tube and into the conical flask containing the limewater.

Results
Limewater turns cloudy or milky showing that carbon dioxide has been evolved.

Conclusion
Yeast ferments the sugar, sucrose to produce carbon dioxide. Alcohol will also be formed.

Sugars

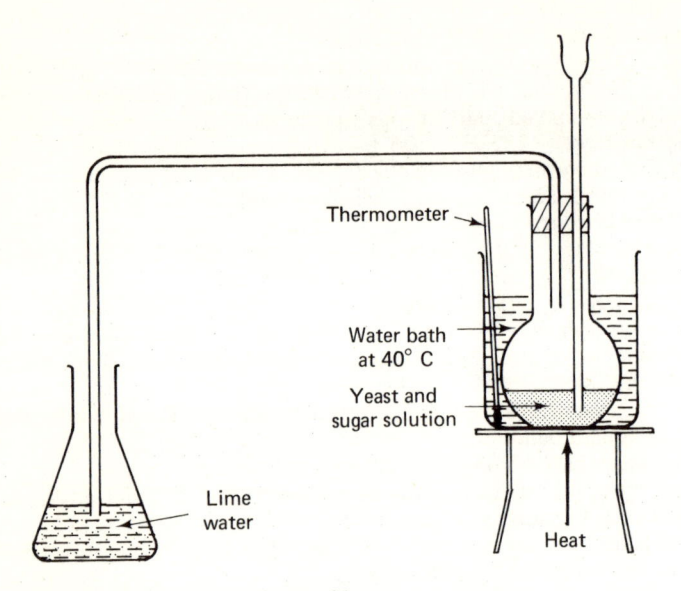

Diagram: apparatus with flask containing yeast and sugar solution in a water bath at 40°C with thermometer, connected via tube to a flask of lime water; heat applied below.

Labels: Thermometer; Water bath at 40° C; Yeast and sugar solution; Lime water; Heat

Experiment to show the effects of heat on cane sugar
Apparatus
    1 test tube   1 bunsen burner
    1 test tube holder   1 spatula
Reagents
Cane sugar
Method
    Place a small amonnt of sugar in a dry test tube and heat over a bunsen burner. Observe changes in colour and consistency.
Results
    Sugar liquifies and gradually becomes darker in colour as the sugar changes into caramel.

14
Fats and Oils

Fats and oils belong to a class of compounds called lipids. Most fats and oils are triglycerides, composed therefore of glycerol and three fatty acids. Fats and oils differ in that fats are solid at room temperature while oils are in the liquid state at room temperature.

Properties of fats and oils
1 All fats and oils are insoluble in water but soluble in organic solvents such as ether and carbon tetrachloride.
2 Melting point. Most fats and oils in foods consist of complex mixtures of triglycerides and therefore they do not have a sharp melting point.
3 Plasticity. Just before their melting point fats become plastic; at this point they are soft and easily spreadable. In any given fat there is generally a mixture of triglycerides and as they have differing melting points some are in the liquid state and some are in the solid state. The triglycerides which are in the solid state form a crystalline network, the liquid triglycerides are present as droplets of oil in between the crystals. The crystals are able to slide on one another giving the fat its plasticity.
   If the fat contains a high proportion of triglycerides in the liquid state the fat will be very plastic and as soon as the temperature is raised the fat quickly becomes an oil. If a fat contains only one type of triglyceride it will not be plastic as it will either be made of crystals or oil.
4 *Smoke point* This is the temperature at which a fat or oil gives off a bluish smoke. The smoke point of lard is 171°C and 210°C for cottonseed oil.
Flash point This is the temperature at which the vapour above the fat or oil will ignite.
Fire point This is the temperature at which the fat or oil will support continued combustion.
5 Rancidity. Most fats and oils do not store well as they develop off flavours and odours. This is known as rancidity. High temperature,

Fats and Oils

presence of moisture, oxygen and light are among the factors which speed up rancidity. There are two types of rancidity, the first type is hydrolytic rancidity caused by the presence of water in which the triglycerides are split into glycerol and three fatty acids. The second type is oxidative rancidity which involves oxygen, the mechanism of the reactions involved is very complex. Antioxidants such as vitamin E are present naturally in many fats and oils and these help to retard rancidity. Commercially antioxidants are added to fats and oils to prolong their shelf life.

6   Iodine number. This is a measure of the degree of unsaturation of the fat or oil. It is the number of grammes of iodine that are absorbed by 100 g of fat or oil. If a fat or oil contains unsaturated fatty acids the double bonds readily take up iodine.

7   Colour of fats. The colour of fats and oils is due to many pigments. The orange and yellow colours are due to the presence of carotenoids.

Commercial sources of fat products

Fats do not occur free in nature but they can readily be extracted from a variety of sources, eg from animal tissues, fruit, seeds and milk.

1   Lard is prepared from the processed fat of hogs.
2   Butter is prepared from cream.
3   Vegetable oils are extracted from cottonseeds, soyabeans, olives, maize, sunflower seeds and groundnut seeds.
4   Marine oils; these are extracted from oily fish and whales, although whale oil is in short supply at present.

Vegetable oils are used as cooking oils. Olive oil is used as a salad dressing. The high proportion of unsaturated fatty acids in the vegetable oils makes them desirable from the dietary angle.

A mixture of vegetable and marine oils is used in the preparation of margarine.

The manufacture of margarine

1   The chosen mixture of oils is purified so that the oils are free from colour and odour.
2   The oils are then neutralised to remove free fatty acids which would oxidise and cause rancidity in a later stage.
3   The oils are hydrogenated. This means that the oils are subjected to hydrogen and some hydrogen is added on to the double bonds of the unsaturated fatty acids making them saturated. As the fatty acids become saturated the oils solidify. Since margarine is in the solid state at room temperature it is necessary to solidify some of the oils.

Hydrogenation

```
    H   H   H   H   H
    |   |   |   |   |
 ---C—C—C = C—C---     Part of an unsaturated
    |   |       |          fatty acid molecule
    H   H       H
                |   Addition of hydrogen in the
                ▼   presence of a nickel catalyst

    H   H   H   H   H
    |   |   |   |   |
 ---C—C—C—C—C---       Part of a saturated
    |   |   |   |   |     fatty acid molecule
    H   H   H   H   H
```

Hydrogenation is never carried out to completion because if all the fatty acids in the oils were completely saturated the margarine would be too hard.
4   The resulting mixture is treated so that the margarine will have a suitable melting point.
5   The mixture is refined again as hydrogenation produces products with an undesirable flavour.
6   The fats are blended so that the margarine will have a suitable consistency, melting point and plasticity.
7   The fats are mixed with ripened or sweet milk to form an emulsion and then the margarine is packed. The margarine usually has salt added to it, also vitamins A and D and colourings such as anatto and carotene. Emulsifiers such as lecithin and monoglycerides and flavouring agents such as butyric acid present in butter are added to the margarine in the final stages of its manufacture.

Cooking fats

These are blends of oils and fats which are used for shortening the gluten in flour confectionery. They are often made from a mixture of palm oil, lard and fish oils. Cooking fats are made entirely of fats and oils whereas margarine is an oil in water emulsion. The oils used in the preparation of a cooking fat are partially hydrogenated and then blended. The mixture is often whipped to incorporate air and the result is the formation of a smooth white solid.

A cooking fat must be plastic, an effective shortener and a good creaming agent.

Uses of fats in cooking

1   Fat gives a desirable flavour to food. Fats act as carriers for many food flavours, eg spices, herbs and vanilla.
2   Fats are used to make emulsions. Fat is naturally present in milk and egg yolk which are emulsions. Fat is used in mayonnaise preparation. Emulsified fat is present in many baked goods.

Fats and Oils

3   Fat is used in frying to prevent food from sticking to the pan; it transfers the heat and gives flavour and colour to the food.
4   Fat traps air in the creaming process of cake-making and so improves the texture. Fat is usually warmed before it is used for creaming to make it plastic, then it is creamed with sugar and air is trapped.
5   Fat shortens the gluten strands in flour confectionery producing products with a short crust, eg shortbread. The fat coats the starch and the gluten in the flour preventing the strands of gluten from joining together. When pastry is made with insufficient fat it is tough because the gluten strands have not been shortened sufficiently.

EXPERIMENTAL STUDY OF FATS AND OILS

EXPERIMENT 1

Determination of the melting point of various fats
Apparatus
    Water bath
    Thermometer
    Rubber band
    Capillary tubes
       (melting point tubes)

    Bunsen burner
    Tripod
    Gauze
    Clamp stand

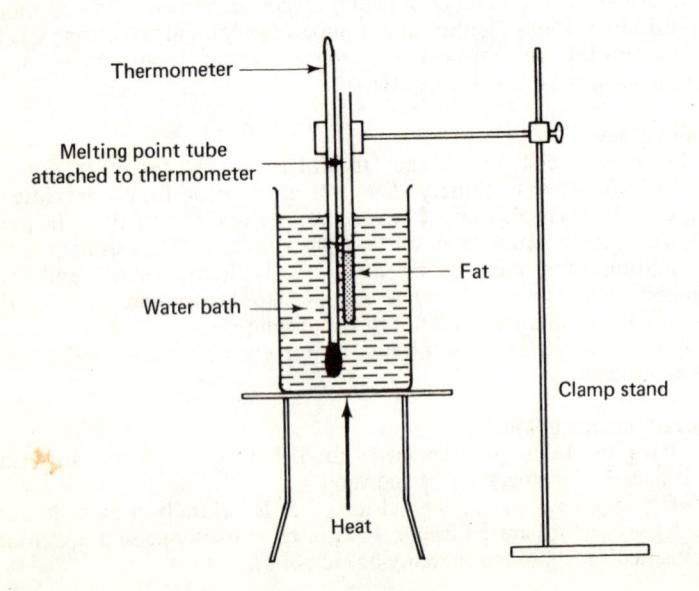

Practical Work

Method
   Place a small amount of the fat to be tested in a capillary tube, seal one end of the tube using the flame of a bunsen burner. Attach the capillary tube to a thermometer and clamp in position in the water bath. Heat the water very slowly until the fat becomes transparent. Note the temperature. Allow the water to cool and then heat the water again to get a second reading for the melting point. Repeat the experiment with other fat samples.

EXPERIMENT 2

Experiment to show the variation in the quality of fried food with the type of fat used
Method
   Prepare some chipped potatoes. Place a small quantity of fat or oil in a frying pan and allow to reach smoke point. Fry 50 g of chips in the hot fat. Note the weight of the chips after cooking. Note also their taste, degree of greasiness, texture, colour, etc. Repeat with different samples of oils and fats.
   Which product produces the most desirable chips?
   Which chips will be the highest in Calorie content?

EXPERIMENT 3

Experiment to show the function of fat in a sponge mix
Basic recipe
   56 g of flour   1 egg
   56 g of fat   ½ dessertspoonful
   56 g of castor sugar   of milk
Method
1   Prepare a sponge in the normal manner using the basic recipe.
2   Prepare a sponge using 28 g of fat instead of 56 g
3   Prepare a sponge using 84 g of fat instead of 56 g
4   Prepare a sponge using 112 g of fat instead of 56 g
5   Prepare a sponge using no fat.
   Describe the texture, flavour and colour of each of the five sponges.

15
Vegetables and Fruits

A great variety of vegetables are eaten in the diet and these are obtained from many different parts of the plant.
Classification of vegetables according to the part of the plant that is eaten
1 *Leaves*
Cabbage, spinach, lettuce, kale, parsley.
2 *Leaf bud*
Brussels sprouts.
3 *Stems*
Celery, asparagus, leeks
4 *Stem and leaf*
Chicory, watercress, mustard and cress.
5 *Roots*
Carrot, turnip, parsnip, beetroot, radish, swede.
6 *Tubers*
Potatoes, Jerusalem artichokes
7 *Bulbs*
Onions, shallots, garlic.
8 *Flowers*
Cauliflower, globe artichoke, broccoli.
9 *Fruit*
Runner beans, marrow, cucumber, tomato, aubergine, pumpkin, peppers.
10 *Seeds*
Peas, broad beans, haricot beans, sweetcorn.
11 *Fungi*
Mushrooms.

The nutritional value of vegetables
Water
Water content is generally high. In the case of the marrow the water content is as high as 97.8%.

Nutritional Value of Vegetables

Protein
The green leafy vegetables are low in their protein content, but peas and beans are a good source. The protein present is not of such high quality as that in animal foods but if a variety of vegetables is eaten together as in the vegetarian diet the supplementary effect of amino acids takes place. Soya beans are an exceptionally rich source of vegetable protein.

Carbohydrates
Vegetables usually contain starch and sugar. The leafy vegetables are low in their carbohydrate content, but potatoes, peas and parsnips have quite a high percentage of starch. All vegetables contain the carbohydrate cellulose which is useful in the diet as roughage.

Fats
The fat content of vegetables is unimportant and in the food tables the vegetables are given as containing only a trace of fat.

Minerals
The minerals present in vegetables vary tremendously due to the varying mineral content of the soil. Vegetables usually contain sodium, potassium, calcium, magnesium, iron, copper, phosphorus and sulphur amongst others. The outer leaves of leafy vegetables are a better source of minerals than the inner leaves.

Vitamins
All vegetables contain vitamin C which is very soluble in cooking water and heat labile. Thus great care must be taken in handling vegetables in order to preserve the vitamin C. Many vegetables are good sources of carotene, the precursor of vitamin A, eg carrots and spinach. Vegetables contain some of the B vitamins but do not contain any vitamin D.

A vegetable of special note: the potato
The potato is a unique food in that it contains virtually all the nutrients required for health.

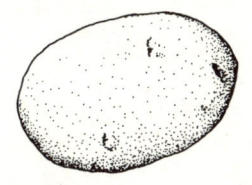

It is very easy to grow and provides a good yield per hectare.
The potato is perhaps not so fattening as many people believe, eg
    100 g of butter produces 793 Calories of energy
    100 g of sugar produces 394 Calories of energy
    100 g of bread produces 243 Calories of energy
    100 g of potato produces 80 Calories of energy

Vegetables and Fruits

As soon as potatoes become chips then the Calorie content increases alarmingly.

	Calories per 100 g
Boiled potatoes	80
Roast potatoes	123
Chipped potatoes	239
Crisps	559

Potatoes are a useful source of vitamin C in the diet. When harvested they contain 30 mg of vitamin C per 100 g. During storage the vitamin C content drops to about 8 mg/100 g in March and after March the vitamin C content will be practically nil. If the potato is peeled and boiled 30-50% of the vitamin C is lost and if the potatoes are kept warm for two hours before serving the vitamin C content is reduced by a further 50%. Thus potatoes that have been stored until March and then boiled and kept hot for two hours will contain about 2 mg of vitamin C per 100 g. The average daily consumption of potatoes in this country is about 160 g per head, thus the vitamin C obtained from the daily portion of boiled new potatoes could be between 24 and 32 mg.

Instant mashed potatoes can be a good source of vitamin C as leading manufacturers add vitamin C to their product.

FRUITS

Fruits form a class of food which has a pleasant flavour; they are usually juicy and have attractive colours.

They contain a high percentage of water. Fruits also contain sugars, mineral salts and acids such as citric acid in citrus fruits and malic acid in apples. Orange coloured fruits contain carotene. Fruits contain negligible amounts of protein and fat and they do not contain any vitamin D. Dried fruits are useful in the diet for their iron content.

Nutritional value of some common vegetables
Per 100 g edible portion

	Water g	Protein g	Calories	Calcium mg	Iron mg	Vitamin C mg
Beans, broad, boiled	83.7	4.1	43	21.2	0.98	15
Beans, french, boiled	95.5	0.8	7	38.6	0.59	5
Beans, runner, boiled	93.6	0.8	7	25.6	0.59	5
Beetroot, boiled	82.7	1.8	44	30	0.70	5
Brussels sprouts, boiled	90.8	2.4	16	27.1	0.63	35
Broccoli,	90.8	3.1	14	160	1.52	40
Cabbage, boiled	95.0	1.0	8	52	0.6	20
Carrots, young, boiled	81.1	0.9	21	28.8	0.43	4
Cauliflower, boiled	94.9	1.5	11	23	0.48	20
Celery, boiled	95.7	0.6	5	52	0.43	5
Cucumber	96.4	0.6	9	22.8	0.30	8
Leeks, boiled	90.8	1.8	25	60.5	2.0	15
Lettuce	95.2	1.1	11	25.9	0.73	15
Marrow, boiled	97.8	0.4	7	13.6	0.22	2
Mushrooms, raw	91.5	1.8	7	2.9	1.03	3
Onions, boiled	96.6	0.6	13	24.4	0.25	6
Parsnips, boiled	83.2	1.3	56	35.5	0.45	10
Peas, fresh, boiled	80.0	5.0	49	12.6	1.22	15
Potatoes, boiled	80.5	1.4	80	4.3	0.48	4-21*
Spinach, boiled	85.1	5.1	26	595.	4.00	25
Tomatoes	93.4	0.9	14	13.3	0.43	20
Watercress	91.1	2.9	15	222	1.62	60

* depending on storage time

Nutritional value of some common fruits
Per 100 g edible portion

	Water g	Calories	Available carbohydrate g	Carotene mg	Vitamin C mg
Apples	84.5	45	11.7	0.03	5
Apricots, fresh	86.6	28	6.7	1.5	7
Apricots, dried	71.6	61	14.4	1.2	Trace
Bananas	70.7	77	19.2	0.2	10
Blackberries	82.0	30	6.4	0.1	20
Cherries	81.5	47	11.9	0.12	5
Currants, black	77.4	29	6.6	0.2	200
Currants, red	82.8	21	4.4		40
Canned fruit salad	77.6	70	18.5	0.30	3
Gooseberries	89.9	17	3.4	0.18	40
Grapes	80	60	16.0	Trace	4
Grapefruit	90.7	22	5.3	Trace	40
Lemons, whole	85.2	15	3.2	0	50
Melons, yellow	94.2	21	5.0	2.0	25
Oranges	86.1	35	8.5	0.05	50
Peaches	86.2	37	9.1	0.50	8
Pears	83.4	40	10.4	0.01	3
Pineapple	84.3	46	11.6	0.06	25
Plums, dessert	85.1	38	9.6	0.22	3
Prunes, stewed	61.6	81	20.2	0.50	Trace
Raspberries	83.2	25	5.6	0.08	25
Rhubarb, stewed	95.5	5	0.8	0.05	7
Strawberries	88.9	26	6.2	0.03	60

NUTS

Nuts are useful in the diet for their protein, calcium, fat and carbohydrate content. They are invaluable in the diet of vegetarians and vegans.

Nutritional value of some common nuts
per 100 g edible portion

	Calories	*Protein g*	*Fat g*	*Carbohydrate g*	*Calcium mg*
Almonds	598	20.5	53.5	4.3	247
Brazil nuts	644	13.8	61.5	4.1	176
Chestnuts	172	2.3	2.7	36.6	46
Coconut	365	3.8	36.0	3.7	13
Peanuts	603	28.1	49.0	8.6	61
Walnuts	549	12.5	51.5	5.0	61

The structure of fruits and vegetables
All fruits and vegetables consist of a vast number of plant cells which have large vacuoles and a cellulose cell wall.

A typical plant cell

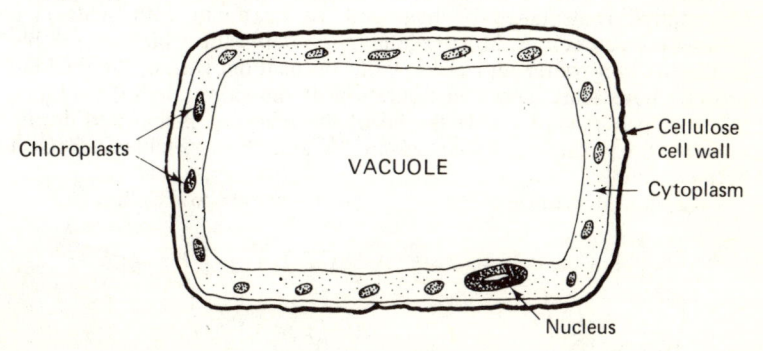

Vegetables and Fruits

The vacuole contains the cell sap which consists of water, minerals, soluble vitamins, colloidally dispersed proteins, sugar, a trace of fat and enzymes.

The chloroplasts contain chlorophyll and thus carry out the process of photosynthesis. They also contain other pigments such as carotenoids.

Leucoplasts are starch containing bodies present in the cytoplasm of starchy vegetables.

The cell wall is made of cellulose and some pectin. In older plants lignin is present in the cell walls making the fruit or vegetable woody.

Pectin is found in between the plant cells. There is a large amount of pectin in apples and citrus fruits.

Effect of cooking on the structure of plant cells

The cellulose cell wall softens on cooking making the fruit or vegetable more palatable and digestible. The amount of cellulose in a vegetable determines its cooking time, eg spinach contains very little cellulose and so cooks quickly and carrots contain a high proportion of cellulose and so require a long cooking time.

The pectin in the intercellular spaces dissolves during cooking and this separates the cells. The air in the intercellular spaces is forced out and the cell contents coagulate due to the effect of heat. Any starch present will gelatinise in the presence of heat and water.

Alkaline cooking water makes vegetables soft and slimy. The alkaline medium speeds up the destruction of vitamin C. The advantage of putting an alkali such as bicarbonate of soda in the cooking water is to preserve the colour. Acid cooking water tends to make vegetables tough. The acid environment will help to preserve vitamin C but tends to break down the chlorophyll and produce vegetables with a poor colour.

Plant pigments

Chlorophyll

This is the green pigment found in the leaves and stems of plants. Chlorophyll is degraded by heat and by treatment with acids to a yellowish-green colour. Most vegetables contain acids which are soluble in the cooking water and are volatile on heating. During the cooking process these acids cause discolouration of the chlorophyll if the lid of the saucepan is kept on. If the lid of the saucepan is removed during cooking the volatile acids are given off and the vegetables will be a better colour.

Volatile acids escaping   Volatile acids trapped by lid

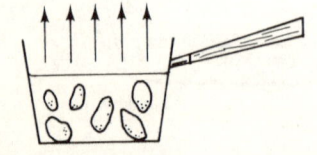

Anthocyanins
These are red pigments present in beetroot, rhubarb and red cabbage. In an acid medium the colour of anthocyanins is enhanced, while in an alkaline medium the red colour becomes a greyish-blue colour.
Carotenoids
These compounds are responsible for the colour of orange and yellow fruits and vegetables such as apricots and carrots. Carotenoids are little affected by acids, alkalis or heat. They are present in plants in conjunction with chlorophyll. If the orange coloured vegetable or fruit is in an acid medium the chlorophyll colour is partially destroyed and the colour of the carotenoid therefore becomes brighter.
Flavones (Anthoxanthins)
These are present in white vegetables and fruits. They are sensitive to pH; in an acid medium they are white but in an alkaline medium they are yellow.

Summary of pigments

	Colour in acid medium	*Colour in alkaline medium*	*Effect of heat*
Chlorophyll	Yellow-green	Bright green	Degraded
Anthocyanins	Red	Grey-blue	Unaffected
Carotenoids	Orange-yellow	Orange-yellow	Unaffected
Flavones	White	Yellow	Unaffected

Browning reactions
Enzymic browning occurs in fruits and vegetables when the cells are cut or bruised. The probable mechanism is that copper containing enzymes are released when the cells are broken and they act on phenol compounds present in the fruit or vegetable producing a brown colour. When vegetables are blanched before freezing these browning enzymes are destroyed. Fruits and vegetables with a high concentration of phenols and browning enzymes brown readily, eg apples, peaches, potatoes, bananas, grapes and cherries.
Fruit and vegetables with a low concentration of phenols or browning enzymes do not turn brown readily, eg citrus fruits, raspberries, blackberries, tomatoes and melons.

Prevention of browning
Browning can be prevented by using acids, eg adding lemon juice to bananas. Vitamin C (ascorbic acid) is also effective. Sulphur dioxide is

commonly used to prevent browning.

If potatoes are placed under water then this temporarily prevents browning. Solutions of sugar and salt have the same effect as they prevent oxygen from the atmosphere coming into contact with the plant cells.

Compounds such as potassium metabisulphite and citric acid are used commercially to prevent browning. Cooking and blanching destroy the enzymes that cause browning.

EXPERIMENTAL WORK ON FRUITS AND VEGETABLES
Experiment to investigate the prevention of browning in fruits and vegetables

Take a selection of fruits and vegetables; prepare and cut into small pieces. Place a sample of each of the fruits and vegetables on a saucer, note time taken by each sample to turn brown. Place further samples of the fruits and vegetables on saucers and add a few millilitres of the following solutions to each type of fruit and vegetable. Note the time taken for browning to occur in each case.

1 Tap water
2 Distilled water
3 3% sugar solution
4 3% salt solution
5 3% citric acid solution
6 3% vitamin C solution
7 3% potassium metabisulphite solution
8 Lemon juice
9 Vinegar
10 3% sodium bicarbonate solution

Which solution is the most effective in the prevention of browning?

Experiment to compare samples of pectin extracted from various fruits
Apparatus
   3 beakers
   1 Buchner funnel attached to flask with a side arm leading to pump on tap
   1 pestle and mortar
   1 200 ml measuring cylinder
   1 electrically heated water bath

Reagents
   pH paper
   Dilute hydrochloric acid
   Methylated spirits
   Filter paper

Method
Obtain samples of various fruits, eg citrus fruits, apples, pears, plums, cherries, strawberries. Grind 50 g of sample with a pestle and mortar to make a pulp. Add dilute hydrochloric acid to the pulp until its pH is about 2. Test the pH using pH paper. Boil pulp gently for about 15 minutes. Filter under pressure through a Buchner funnel. Place filtrate obtained in a beaker containing 200 ml of methylated spirits. Pectin separates as a gel. Evaporate off the methylated spirits using a water bath. Repeat the experiment with different fruits and compare the pectin samples obtained.

Practical Work

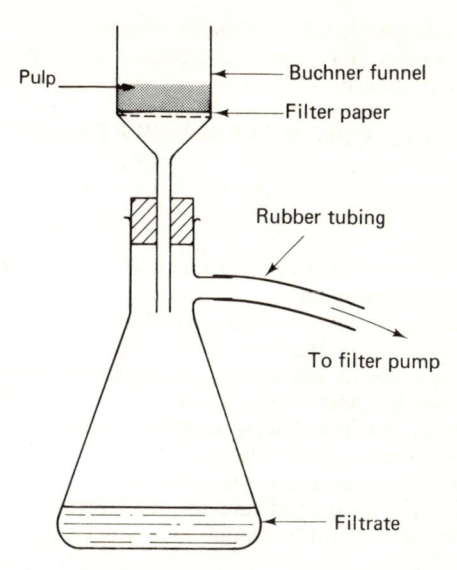

```
Pulp ──→ ▓▓▓▓  ←── Buchner funnel
         ─────  ←── Filter paper
                ── Rubber tubing
                ── To filter pump
                ── Filtrate
```

Which sample gives the firmest gel? Which fruit will set most readily in jam making?

EXPERIMENTAL COOKING OF CABBAGE
Standard
Add 100 g of prepared cabbage to a small measured quantity of boiling salted water in a saucepan with a lid. Start the stopwatch and remove samples after 1, 3, 5, 7, 9, 11 and 20 minutes. Examine samples and decide on the optimum cooking time.

Variants
In each case use 100 g of prepared cabbage in the same quantity of water used above and cook each sample for the optimum time.
1   Add 1 teaspoonful of vinegar to the cooking water.
2   Add 2 teaspoonsful of vinegar to the cooking water.
3   Add a pinch of bicarbonate of soda to the cooking water.
4   Add 1 teaspoonful of bicarbonate of soda to the cooking water.
5   Cook the cabbage with the lid of the saucepan removed.
Note colour, flavour and texture of the cabbage in each case.

Results
1   Cabbage is tough and has an olive green colour.
2   Cabbage is very tough, tastes of vinegar and has a pale colour.
3   Cabbage has a bright green colour but it is soft.
4   Cabbage has a very bright colour but is very soft and slimy.

Vegetables and Fruits

5   Colour is better than that of the standard.
   This experiment illustrates the effect of varying pH on the colour and texture of cabbage.

EXPERIMENTAL WORK ON VEGETABLE PIGMENTS

Anthocyanins

Experiment 1
1   Take a sample of red cabbage and soak it in water for 30 minutes. Strain and retain the liquid.
2   Cook a sample of red cabbage in boiling water for 20 minutes. Strain and retain the liquid.
3   Cook a sample of red cabbage in boiling water which has 2 teaspoonsful of vinegar added to it. Strain and retain the liquid.
4   Repeat (3) but add 2 teaspoonsful of sodium bicarbonate to the cooking water instead of the vinegar.
   Note pH and colour of the 4 samples of liquid. Note flavour, texture and colour of the 4 samples of cabbage. What effect does pH have on the colour of the pigment anthocyanin?

Experiment 2
   Take 3 portions of diced beetroot. To the first portion add some vinegar, to the second portion add distilled water and to the third portion add some sodium bicarbonate solution.
Results
   The vinegar brightens the colour of the beetroot. The alkaline sodium bicarbonate solution makes the anthocyanin in the beetroot a greyish-purple colour.

Flavones

Experiment
   Cook some onions in acid, alkaline and neutral solutions and note how the flavone which is the white pigment, changes colour.

Carotenoids

Experiment
   Cook some carrots in neutral, acid and alkaline cooking water. Note their colour after cooking.

Results
   Carotenoids are not affected by changes in pH.

The estimation of vitamin C in fruits and vegetables
Principle

Vitamin C is extracted from the food source by grinding it with an acid mixture and sand. The vitamin C extract is titrated against indophenol dye which oxidises ascorbic acid to dehydroascorbic acid. The blue dye turns pink as it comes into contact with the acid mixture used to extract the vitamin C. The vitamin C bleaches the dye. The end point of the titration is when a pale pink colour is present for 10 seconds or more. At the end point just enough dye has been added to react with all the vitamin C so there is no vitamin C left to bleach the dye and the pale pink colour is seen.

Apparatus
- 100 ml burette
- 1 screw top jar
- 3 conical flasks
- Pestle and mortar
- Muslin
- 1 glass funnel
- 2 100 ml flasks
- 1 5 ml pipette
- 1 20 ml measuring cylinder

Reagents

Acid mixture made with 15 g of metaphosphoric acid 40 ml of glacial acetic acid and 400 ml of distilled water
Sand
Food sample
Dichlorophenolindophenol dye tablets which have a titration value equivalent to 1 mg of vitamin C.

Method

1 Take 1 dichlorophenolindophenol tablet and grind it with a pestle and mortar, add distilled water and transfer contents of the mortar into a 100 ml flask. Wash out the mortar with distilled water and transfer washings to the flask. Make up to the 100 ml mark with distilled water. Transfer the dye to the burette.

2 Put 15 ml of the acid mixture in the screw top jar.

3 Weigh out a 5 g sample of the food sample, place in the screw top jar and shake.

4 Transfer contents of the jar to a mortar and grind with sand.

5 Filter the liquid through the muslin in a glass funnel into a 100 ml flask.

6 Add 10 ml of the acid mixture to the solid remaining in the mortar and grind.

7 Filter contents of the mortar through the muslin into the 100 ml flask. Wash the mortar with distilled water and again filter through the muslin. Wash residue in the muslin with distilled water, collect the washings and make the volume of liquid in the flask up to 100 ml with distilled water. This flask then contains the vitamin C from the food sample in a solution of known volume. Vitamin C is stable in an acid environment.

Vegetables and Fruits

8   Pipette 5 ml portions of the vitamin C solution into the conical flasks.

9   Add the dye from the burette to the vitamin C solution in a conical flask drop by drop until a pale pink colour persists for 10 seconds. Note the volume of dye used. Repeat titration with other 5 ml portions of vitamin C solution until 2 very close results are obtained.

Sample calculation

Supposing the average volume of dye used in the titrations is 12 ml.

ie   100 ml of dye ≡ 1 mg of Vitamin C.

∴ 12 ml of dye ≡ 1 x $\frac{12}{100}$ mg of Vit C.

Thus a 5 ml portion of the Vitamin C solution contains

$$1 \times \frac{12}{100} \text{ mg of Vit C.}$$

Therefore the 100 ml solution of Vitamin C contains

$$1 \times \frac{12}{100} \times \frac{100}{5} \text{ mg of Vitamin C.}$$

Thus the 5 g portion of the food contained $1 \times \frac{12}{100} \times \frac{100}{5}$ mg of Vit C.

It is usual to express the Vit C content per 100 g of the food sample

So Vit C content of 100 g of food = $1 \times \frac{12}{100} \times \frac{100}{5} \times \frac{100}{5}$

= 48 mg of Vit C.

Using this method the vitamin C content of 100 g of food can be obtained by multiplying the volume of dye used in the titration by 4.

NB This method for the estimation of vitamin C is not suitable for foods with a strong colour as the colour masks the pale pink end point.

Useful experiments can be made using this method to compare the vitamin C values of foods which have been cooked or preserved in various ways, eg fresh and tinned grapefruit, baked, boiled and chipped potatoes, potato powder and canned potatoes, raw and cooked cabbage, the cooking water could also be tested, fresh, canned, frozen canned and dehydrated orange juice.

Overleaf
Table showing
**Recommended Daily Intakes
of Energy and Nutrients
for the UK (1969)**

RECOMMENDED DAILY INTAKES OF

Age Range	Occupational category	Body weight kg	Energy kcal	Energy MJ	Protein g
BOYS AND GIRLS					
0 up to 1 year		7.3	800	3.3	20
1 up to 2 years		11.4	1200	5.0	30
2 up to 3 years		13.5	1400	5.9	35
3 up to 5 years		16.5	1600	6.7	40
5 up to 7 years		20.5	1800	7.5	45
7 up to 9 years		25.1	2100	8.8	53
BOYS					
9 up to 12 years		31.9	2500	10.5	63
12 up to 15 years		45.5	2800	11.7	70
15 up to 18 years		61.0	3000	12.6	75
GIRLS					
9 up to 12 years		33.0	2300	9.6	58
12 up to 15 years		48.6	2300	9.6	58
15 up to 18 years		56.1	2300	9.6	58
MEN					
18 up to 35 years	Sedentary	65	2700	11.3	68
	Moderately active		3000	12.6	75
	Very active		3600	15.1	90
35 up to 65 years	Sedentary	65	2600	10.9	65
	Moderately active		2900	12.1	73
	Very active		3600	15.1	90
65 up to 75 years	Assuming a	63	2350	9.8	59
75 and over	sedentary life	63	2100	8.8	53
WOMEN					
18 up to 55 years	Most occupations	55	2200	9.2	55
	Very active		2500	10.5	63
55 up to 75 years	Assuming a	53	2050	8.6	51
75 and over	sedentary life	53	1900	8.0	48
Pregnancy, 2nd and 3rd trimester			2400	10.0	60
Lactation			2700	11.3	68

ENERGY AND NUTRIENTS FOR THE UK (1969)
Department of Health and Social Security

Thiamine	Ribo-flavine	Nicotinic acid	Ascorbic acid	Vitamin A	Vitamin D	Calcium	Iron
mg	mg	mg equiva-lents	mg	μg retinol equiv-alents	μg cholecal-ciferol	mg	mg
0.3	0.4	5	15	450	10	600	6
0.5	0.6	7	20	300	10	500	7
0.6	0.7	8	20	300	10	500	7
0.6	0.8	9	20	300	10	500	8
0.7	0.9	10	20	300	2.5	500	8
0.8	1.0	11	20	400	2.5	500	10
1.0	1.2	14	25	575	2.5	700	13
1.1	1.4	16	25	725	2.5	700	14
1.2	1.7	19	30	750	2.5	600	15
0.9	1.2	13	25	575	2.5	700	13
0.9	1.4	16	25	725	2.5	700	14
0.9	1.4	16	30	750	2.5	600	15
1.1	1.7	18	30	750	2.5	500	10
1.2	1.7	18	30	750	2.5	500	10
1.4	1.7	18	30	750	2.5	500	10
1.0	1.7	18	30	750	2.5	500	10
1.2	1.7	18	30	750	2.5	500	10
1.4	1.7	18	30	750	2.5	500	10
0.9	1.7	18	30	750	2.5	500	10
0.8	1.7	18	30	750	2.5	500	10
0.9	1.3	15	30	750	2.5	500	12
1.0	1.3	15	30	750	2.5	500	12
0.8	1.3	15	30	750	2.5	500	10
0.7	1.3	15	30	750	2.5	500	10
1.0	1.6	18	60	750	10	1200	15
1.1	1.8	21	60	1200	10	1200	15

reproduced by courtesy of the Controller of Her Majesty's Stationary Office

Bibliography

USEFUL NUTRITION BOOKS

ELEMENTARY AND INTERMEDIATE LEVELS

GENERAL TEXTBOOKS
The Value of Food, P. Fisher and A. Bender, *Oxford University Press*
Nutrition and Elementary Food Science, H. Marks, *Warne*
The Manual of Nutrition, Ministry of Agriculture Fisheries and Food, *HMSO*
Food and Nutrition, W.M. Rankin and E.M. Hildreth, *Allman*
Second Book of Food and Nutrition, W. Matthews and D. Wells, *Forbes*
Nutrition for Practical Nurses, Have, *Saunders*
Dietetic Foods, A. Bender, *Leonard Hill*

SPECIAL TOPICS
Wheat in Human Nutrition, W. Ackroyd and J. Doughty, *FAO*
Legumes in Human Nutrition, W. Ackroyd and J. Doughty, *FAO*
Eating to Live, D. Wells, *Times Newspapers*
This Slimming Business, J. Yudkin, *Penguin Books*
Food, Facts and Fallacies, A. G. Cameron, *Faber*
Synthetic Food, M. Pyke, *Murray*
Technological Eating, M. Pyke, *Murray*

FOOD TABLES
The Composition of Foods, R. McCance and E. Widdowson, *HMSO*

Dictionary of Nutrition and Food Technology, A. Bender, *Butterworth*

BOOKLETS AND JOURNALS
Getting the Most out of Food, Series of booklets available from *Van den Berghs*
Nutrition Information Booklets from the *British Nutrition Foundation* (Alembic House, 93, Albert Embankment, London SE1)

Bibliography

Home Economics
Housecraft
Quarterly Review of Nutrition and Food Science
Nutrition
Household Food Consumption and Expenditure (National Food Survey), Ministry of Agriculture, Fisheries and Food. *HMSO*

ADVANCED GENERAL TEXTBOOKS
Human Nutrition and Dietetics, S. Davidson and R. Passmore, *Livingstone* (an excellent Nutrition reference book)
Hutchison's Food and the Principles of Nutrition, H. Sinclair and D. Hollingsworth, *Arnold*
Cooper's Nutrition in Health and Disease, 15th Edition, Mitchell, Rynbergen, Anderson and Dibble, *Pitman Medical Publications*
Modern Nutrition in Health and Disease, Wohl and Goodhart, *Lea and Febiger*

SPECIAL TOPICS
Trace Elements in Human and Animal Nutrition, E.J. Underwood, *Academic Press*
The Vitamins in Health and Disease, J. Marks, *Churchill*
Sugar, Yudkin, Edelman and Hough, *Butterworth*
Food Resources, Conventional and Novel, N.W. Pirie, *Penguin Books*
Nutritional Deficiencies in Modern Society, N. Howard and I McLean Baird, *Newman*
World Population and Food Supply, J.H. Lowry, *Arnold*
Food Microbiology, W.C. Frazier, *McGraw Hill*
Pure White and Deadly (sugar) J. Yudkin, *Davis-Poynter*
Micronutrients, *Unilever booklets*
The Chemistry of Proteins, *Unilever booklets*

USEFUL FOOD SCIENCE BOOKS
Elementary and Intermediate
GENERAL TEXTBOOKS
Food Science, B.A. Fox and A.G. Cameron, *University of London Press*
Introductory Food Science, Smith and Walters, *Classic Publications*
Food Science and Technology, M. Pyke, *Murray*
Food Science, Nuffield Advanced Science, *Penguin*
Food Chemistry, L.H. Meyer, *Chapman and Hall*
Experimental Work in Food Science, J.R. Salfield, *Heinemann*

SPECIAL TOPICS
The Oxford Book of Food Plants, *Oxford University Press*
Understanding Cooking, V. Cescrani, *Arnold*
Facts about Margarine, *Van den Berghs*

Bibliography

BOOKLETS
Vegetable Oils and Fats
Margarine and Cooking Fats
Food Preservation: *Unilever series*

ADVANCED GENERAL TEXTBOOKS
The Experimental Study of Foods, R. Griswold, *Constable*
Experimental Cookery, B. Lowe, *Wiley*
Food Theory and Applications, Paul and Palmer, *Wiley*
Principles of Food Science, Vol 1, G. Borgstrom, *Macmillan*

SPECIAL TOPICS
Egg Science and Technology, Stadelman and Cotterill, *AVI Publishing Company*
By-Products from Milk, Well and Whittier, *AVI Publishing Company*
A Dictionary of Dairying, J. Davis, *L. Hill*
Meat Technology, F. Gerrard, *L. Hill*
Meat Science, R.A. Lawrie, *Pergamon*
Modern Cereal Chemistry, D. Kent-Jones and A. Amos, *Food Trade Press*
Technology of Cereals, N.L. Kent, *Pergamon*
Fruit and Vegetables, R.B. Duckworth, *Pergamon*

FILMS

Outline of Slimming, Film Library, Box 68, 2 Kingscote St, London EC4P 4BQ

UNILEVER FILMS
What is Margarine
Nothing to Eat but Food
Bacteria
Food Preservation
Your Digestion

GUILD SOUND AND VISION
Calories and Protein
Pounds, Slimming and Sense
Mineral Elements and Vitamins

NATIONAL AUDIO VISUAL AIDS LIBRARY
Osmosis

FLOUR ADVISORY BUREAU
Protein and Health (an excellent film showing the protein deficiency disease — Kwashiorkor)

ANATOMICAL MODELS

A wide range of anatomical models can be obtained from Griffin and George Ltd (School Suppliers) Ealing Road, Alperton, Wembley, Middlesex HAO 1HJ

VICKERS MICROSCOPES

John H Bassett and Sons, 1 Joule Road, Houndmills Industrial Estate, Basingstoke, Hampshire

Index

Numbers in italics refer to diagrams and tables

Acetic acid 161
Acid calcium phosphate 126, 132
Acidity 19, 20
Acids 20
Actin 113
Adipose tissue 26
Adrenal gland 76
Adrenalin 37
Agar 54
Air 12
Alanine 44
Albumen 113
Alcohol 128, 143
 — energy value 35
Aleurone layer *124*, 125
Alimentary canal 22
Alkalinity 19, 20
Alkalis 20
Alum 29
Aluminium 12
Almonds *52, 74, 75, 80, 155*
Amino acids 12, 25, 27, 28, *31*, 43, 44
Ammonia 28
Amylase 23, 24, 25, 29, *31*, 53, 128
Amylopectin *135*
Amylose *134*
Anaemia 67, 68, 77, 78, 79
Anatto 147
Anthocyanin 157, 160
Anthoxanthin 157
Antioxidant 146
Anus 22, 29
Appendix 22
Apples *39, 45, 61, 69, 86, 154*
Apricots *59, 65, 80, 154*
Arachidlonic acid 51
Arginine 44
Ariboflavinosis 64
Arrowroot *135*
Ascorbic acid 68, 156

Asparagus 150
Aspartic acid 44
Atoms 11
Aubergine 150
Avidin 101

Bacon *39, 52, 64, 66, 76, 80, 114, 116*
Baked beans *39, 80*
Baking powder 132
Bananas 20, *39, 65, 69, 86, 154*
Barley *121, 122,* 123
Basal Metabolic Rate *36*, 39, 81
Beef *39, 45, 52, 66, 68, 74, 80, 86, 114, 116*
Beef corned *80*
Beer *39*
Beetroot 150, *153*
Beri-beri 62, 63
Bicarbonate of soda 20
Bile 24
Bile duct *22, 24*
Biotin 101
Biscuits *39*
Biuret test 55, 88
Blackberries *69, 154*
Black treacle *80*
Body surface area *35*, 36
Bolus 23
Bomb calorimeter *34*
Bones 72, 83
Bovril *76, 80*
Bran 121, *124*
Brazil nuts *155*
Bread *41, 44, 45, 61, 64, 65, 66, 74, 75, 76, 80, 82,* 127
Break rollers 126
Broad beans 150, *153*
Broccoli *74,* 150, *153*
Browning reactions 157
Brussels sprouts 150, *153*
Butter *18, 19, 20, 39, 45, 51, 52,*

170

Index

59, 60, 61, 80, 86, 94-96, 146
Butterscotch *142*
Butyric acid 50, 51, 147

Cabbage 62, 69, 74, 86, 150, *153*, 159
Caecum 22
Cake *39*
Calcium 12, 60, *72*-74
Calcium carbonate 12, 74
Calcium oxalate 78
Calcium phosphate 73
Calorie 33, 36, 39, 40, 41
— allowances 38
Caproic acid 51
Caramel 142, 144
Carbohydrates 11, 12, 28, *31*, 35, 52-55, 63
Carbon *11*, 12, 43, 49, 50, 51, 52
Carbon dioxide *11*, 32, 33, 132
Carotene 58, 59, 147
Carotenoids 113, 146, 157, 160
Carrots 20, *59*, 150, *153*
Casein 88
Caseinogen 88
Cassava 45, 47, 55
Cauliflower 150, *153*
Celery 150, *153*
Cellulose 12, 29, 33, 46, 52, 54, *136*
Cereals 45, 121-133
Cheese *39*, 44, *45*, *52*, *59*, *60*, *64*, *65*, *74*, *75*, *76*, *80*, *86*, *96*, *97*
Chemical changes *14*, *15*
Cherries *154*
Chestnuts *155*
Chicken *39*, *45*, *66*, *80*, *116*
Chicory 150
Chlorine *11*, 72
Chlorine dioxide 126
Chlorophyll 32, 77, 139, 156
Chloroplasts 156
Chocolate *39*, *45*, *52*, *65*, *77*, *80*, 83
Cholecalciferol 60
Cholesterol 49, 51, 101
Chylomicrons 24
Chyme 24

Chymotrypsinogen 25
Citric acid 158
Citrus fruit 68
Cobalt 83
Cocoa *45*
Coconut *80*, *155*
Cod *39*, *45*, *66*, *68*, *86*, 118
Cod liver oil *59*, *60*
Collagen 68, 113
Colloids *18*
Compounds 12
Conalbumen 101
Condensed milk 90
Connective tissue *112*, 113
Continuous phase 18
Cooking fat 147
Cooking oil 146
Copper 12, 83
Copper oxide 30
Copper sulphate 12
Cornflakes *39*
Cottage cheese 96
Cream *18*, *39*, *45*, 93
Cream of tartar 132
Cucumber 150, *153*
Currants — black *69*, *154* — red 154
Curry powder *80*
Cyanocobalamin 67
Cysteine 44
Cystine 44

Deamination 28
Denaturation 104
Dental caries 54, 60, 82
Dermatitis 65
Dextrin *15*, 52, 54
Dextrose *53*
Dichlorophenolindophenol 161
Diffusion 17
Digestion 22-31
Disaccharides 52, 53, 138
Disperse phase 18
Dough 128
Dried milk 89
Duodenum *22*, *24*, 25, *31*
Dyox 126

171

Index

Eggs *39,* 44, *45,* 49, *59,* 60, *61,*
   62, *65, 68, 74, 75, 76, 80, 82,*
   86, 99-111, *114*
— digestion of 31
Egg custard 104
Egg white foam *18,* 104, 107
Egg yolk *18,* 101, 102, 103
Ehrlich's haemotoxylin 118
Eijkman 62
Elastin 113
Elements 12
Emulsions *18,* 19, *88,* 93, 94, 104, 147
Emulsification 24
Emulsifying agent 19
Endomysium *112*
Endosperm *124,* 125
Energy 28, 32-42
Enterogastrone 52
Enterokinase 25
Enzymes 31
Epimysium *112*
Essential amino acids 43-44
Essential fatty acids 41, 51, 52
Ethanol *128*
Evaporated milk 90
Extraction rate of flour 126

Faeces 28
Fats 11, 12, 19, 25, 26, 27, 28, *31,* 35, 49-52, 113, 145-149
Fatty acids 12, 25, 26, 27, *31,* 49, 50, 145
Fehling's test 30, 57, 141
Fermentation 141, 143
Ferritin 78
Ferrous sulphide 103
Fire point of fats 145
Fish *64, 114,* 116-118
Flash point of fats 145
Flavones 123, 157, 160
Flour 64, 125-127
Fluorine 82, 83
Foams *18*
Folic acid 67
Fondant 142

Food calorimeter 40
French beans *86, 153*
Fructose 24, 25, 26, *53,* 54, 57, 138
Fruits 152, 154
Fudge 142

Galactose 25, 26, *53,* 138
Gall bladder *22,* 23, *24*
Garlic 150
Gastric juice 23, 24, *31*
Gel 137
Gelatine *15,* 113, 115
Gelatinisation *15,* 135, 136
Germ *124*
Ginger *80*
Globe artichoke 150
Globulin 113
Glucose 24, 25, 26, *53,* 54, 55, 57, 113, 138
Glutamic acid 44
Gluten 125, 126, 131, 147, 148
Glycerine 50
Glycerol 12, 25, 26, 27, *31, 49,* 50, 145
Glycine 43, 44
Glycogen *26,* 52, 54, 113, 117
Goitre 81-82
Gooseberries *154*
Grapefruit *19, 69,* 154
Grapes *154*
Grass 33

Haddock 76, *82, 118*
Haemoglobin 24, 78, 79
Haemosiderin 78
Ham *76, 114, 116*
Haricot beans 150, *74*
Hepatic portal vein *26, 28*
Herring*39, 59, 60, 68, 80, 82, 118*
Histidine 43
Homogenised milk 89
Horseradish 69
Hydrochloric acid 12, 23, 24, 79
Hydrogen *11,* 12, 43, 49, 50, 51, 52
Hydrogenation of oils *147*
Hydroxyproline 44

172

Index

Hypervitaminosis A, 59
Hypervitaminosis D, 61

Ice *14*
Ice cream 98
Icing 142
Improving agents 126
Insulin 25, 29
Internal respiration 33
Intestinal flora 62
Intestinal juice *21*, 25, 30
Intrinsic factor 23, 67
Inulin 52
Iodine 12, 81, 82, 134
Iodine number 146
Iodine solution 29, 57
Iron 12, 43, 68, 69, *72*, 77-81
Isoleucine 43

Jelly *15, 18*
Jerusalem artichoke 150
Joule 33, 34

Kale 150
Kidneys 28
Kidney (as a food) *59*, 83
Kilocalorie 33
Kilojoule 34, *36*, 38, 41
Kippers *118*
Koilonychia 78
Kwashiorkor 47, 77

Lactalbumen 88, 89
Lactase 25, *31*
Lacteal 26
Lactic acid 20, 63, 113, 117
Lactobacillus acidophilus 98
Lactobacillus bulgaricus 98
Lactoglobulin 88, 89
Lactosazone test 88
Lactose 20, 25, 53, *54*, 57, 88, 138
Lard *39*, 51, *52*, 146
Large intestine *22*
Lauric acid 51
Lead 12
Lecithin 19, 24, 49, 88, 101, 104, 147

Leeks 150, *153*
Legumes 45
Lemons 20, *69, 154*
Lentils *80*
Lettuce *59, 69*, 150, *153*
Leucine 43
Leucoplasts 134, 156
Limiting amino acids 44
Lind James 68
Linoleic acid 51
Linolenic acid 51
Lipase 24, *25*, 26, *31*
Lipids 145
Litmus test 20
Liquorice Allsorts *80*
Liver *22*, 23, 24, 26, 28, 37, 44, 54
Liver (as a food) *59*, 60, *61, 62,
    64, 65, 66, 68, 69, 80, 83, 116*
Loganberries *80*
Long Life milk 89
Luncheon meat *116*
Lymphatic vessel *26*
Lysine 43, 44

Mackerel *118*
Magnesium *72*, 77
Maize 45, 55, 65, 66, *121, 122,*
    123, *135*
Malnutrition 43
Maltase 25, *31*, 53
Maltose 23, 25, *53*, 57, 138
Margarine *18, 52, 60*, 146, 147
Marmalade *45*
Marrow *86*, 150, *154*
Marshmallow *18*
Mayonnaise *18*, 19, 104
Meat 20, 112-116
Megajoules 34, 38
Megaloblastic anaemia 67
Melons *69, 154*
Melting point of fat 51, 145, *147*
Mercury 12
Meringues *18*
Metabolism 37
Metals 12
Metaphosphoric acid 161

173

Index

Methionine 43
Metmyoglobin 113
Milk 12, *18*, 20, *39*, *45*, *59*, *64*, *65*, *68*, *69*, *74*, *75*, *76*, *80*, 82-94
Millet *121*, *122*, 124
Milling of wheat 125
Millons reagent 55, 119
Minerals 19, 28, 72-85
Miners' Cramp 76
Mixtures 12
Molasses 139
Molecule 11
Molisch's test 57, 88
Monosaccharides 52, 53, 138
Monosodium glutamate 76
Mouth *22*, 33
Mucin 23
Muscle fibres *112*
Mushrooms *65*, *66*, 150, *154*
Mustard & cress *69*, *80*, 150
Mutton *52*, *61*, *68*, *114*, *116*
Myoglobin 78, 113
Myosin 113
Myristic acid 51

Napthoquinone 62
Niacytin 65, 66
Nightblindness 58
Nitrogen 12, 43
Non-essential amino acids 43, 44
Non-metals 12
Nougat 142
Nuts 155

Oats *121*, *122*, 123
Obesity 41, 43
Oedema 63, 76
Oesophagus *22*, 23
Offal 112
Oils *15*, *19*, 49-52, 145-149
Oleic acid 51
Olive oil 146
Onions 150, *153*
Oranges *39*, *45*, *59*, *64*, *69*, *86*, *154*
Osazone test 57
Osmium tetroxide 56

Osmosis 15, *16*, 17, 29, 141
Osteomalacia 60, 73
Ovalbumen 101
Oxalic acid 73
Oxygen *11*, 12, 32, 33, 43, 49, 52, 78

Palmitic acid 51
Palmitoleic acid 51
Palm oil 147
Pancreas *22*, 23, *24*, 25, 31
Pancreatic juices 25, *31*
Pantothenic acid 65
Papain 114
Parsley *69*, *74*, *80*, 150
Parsnip *69*, *150*, *153*
Partridge *45*
Pasta 128
Pasteurisation 89
Peaches *69*, *80*, *154*
Peanuts *39*, *45*, *64*, *65*, *155*
Pears *20*, *69*, *80*, *154*
Peas *39*, *45*, *61*, *64*, *65*, *69*, *86*, *150*, *153*
Pectin 12, 52, 54, *141*, *156*
Pellagra 65, 66
Peppers 150
Pepsin 23, 24, *31*
Pepsinogen 23
Peptidases 25, *31*
Peptide bond 43
Peptides 25, *31*
Peptones 24, 25, *31*
Perimysium *112*
Peristalsis 23
Pernicious anaemia 67
Phenylalanine 43
Phospholipids 49
Phosphoproteins 101
Phosphorous 12, 43, 60, *72*
Photosynthesis 32, *138*
pH scale 19, *20*, 23
Physical changes *14*, *15*
Phytic acid 73, 79
Pineapple *69*, *154*
Plaice *74*, *118*

174

Index

Plasticity of fats 145
Plums *154*
Polysaccharides 54
Pork *39, 45, 64, 68, 114, 116*
Porphyrin 100
Potassium 12, *72*, 76
Potassium hydrogen tartrate 132
Potassium metabisulphite 158
Potato *39, 55, 64, 66, 69, 80, 86, 135*, 150, *151, 153*
Prawns *118*
Proline 44
Proteins 11, 12, *18*, 19, 24, 27, 28, *31*, 35, 43-48
Protein quality 44
Protein synthesis 44
Proteoses 24, 25, *31*
Prothrombin 62
Prunes 16, *59, 154*
Pumpkin 150
Pyloric sphincter *22*, 24
Pyridoxine 66
Pyruvic acid 63

Quinine 29

Radish 150
Raising agents 132, 133
Rancidity of fats 145
Raspberries *69, 154*
Rectum *22*, 28
Red blood cells 44, 78
Rennet 91
Rennin 12, *31*, 88, 91, 92
Retinol 58
Rhubarb 20, 73, *154*
Riboflavin 64
Rice 45, 55, 63, *121, 122*, 123, *135*
Rickets 60, 78
Rosehip syrup 69
Roux foundation sauce 137
Ruminants 33
Runner beans *45*, 150, *153*
Rust *14*
Rye *121, 122*, 123

Salad dressing *15, 18*
Saliva 23, 24, 29, 31
Salivary gland *22*
Salmon *64, 118*
Salt 29, 75
Sardines *45, 60, 74, 75, 82, 118*
Saturated fatty acids 50, 51
Sausages *39, 45*, 76, *116*
Scurvy 68
Seaweed *82*
Self raising flour 126
Semi-permeable membrane *15*
Semolina 136
Serine 44
Shallots 150
Slimming diet 41
Small intestine *22*, 24, 25, *26*, 44
Smoke point of fats 145
Sodium *11*, 12, *72*, 75, 76
Sodium bicarbonate 12, 20, 75, 126, 132, 158, 159
Sodium carbonate 132
Sodium chloride *11*, 12, 75
Sodium phosphate 75
Solute 16, 18
Solutions 18
Soya beans 32, 45, 48, *74*, 77, 151
Soya flour *39*
Specific Dynamic Action 37
Spinach *62, 65, 73, 74, 75, 82*, 150, *153*
Sponge making 149
Starches 12, *15, 18*, 19, 23, 25, 29, 32, 52, 53, 55, 134-137
Steam *14*
Stearic acid 51
Sterilised milk 89
Steroids 49
Stomach *22*, 23, *24, 31*
Strawberries *69, 154*
Streptococcus thermophilus 98
Sucrase 25, 30, *31*, 128
Sucrose 12, 13, 19, 24, 30, *54*, 138
Suet 51, *52*
Sugar beet 54, 139, *140*
Sugar boiling 142, 143

175

Index

Sugar boiling thermometer *142*
Sugar cane 54, 139, *140*
Sugars 12, 19, 32, *39*, *45*, 52, 54, 138-144
Sulphur 12, 43, *72*
Sulphur dioxide 12
Sulphuric acid 13, 57
Sultanas *64, 80*
Sunlight 32, 60
Supplementary effect of amino acids 44
Suspensions 19
Sweetcorn 150
Swede 150

Takaki 62
Tapioca *135*, 137
Tartaric acid 132
Taste buds 29
Tea 83
Teeth 72
Textured vegetable protein 48, 49
Thiamine 62, 122
Threonine 43
Thrombosis 49, 54
Thyroid gland 81
Thyroxine 37, 82
Tin 12
Toast *15*
Tocopherol 61
Toffee 142
Tomato 20, *39*, *61*, *62*, *69*, *86*, *150, 153*
Tongue *22*
Trace elements 81
Tributyrin 50
Triglycerides *25*, *31*, 49, 145
Trout *118*
Trypsin 25, *31*
Trypsinogen 25
Tryptophan 43, 66
Turnip 150
Tyrosine 44

Unsaturated fatty acids 51
Urea 28

Urea cycle 28
Urine 28

Valine 43, 44
Veal 114
Vegan 46, 74
Vegetable oil 51, 146
Vegetable protein 44
Vegetables 20, 145, 162
Vegetarian 46, 68, 77, 151
Villus *26*, 28
Vinegar *15*, 19, 20, 158, 159
Vitamins 19, 28, 58-71
Vitamin A 58-60
Vitamin B complex 62-68
Vitamin B_1 62-64
Vitamin B_2 64-65
Vitamin B_3 65
Vitamin B_6 66-67
Vitamin B_{12} 67-68
Vitamin C 20, 68, 69, 126, 130
Vitamin C estimation 161
Vitamin D 60-61
Vitamin E 61
Vitamin K 62
Vitelline membrane *100*, 102

Walnuts *52, 155*
Water *11*, 12, *14*, 20, 28, 32, 33, 84, 86
Watercress *59*, *69*, *80*, 150, *153*
Waterglass 103
Wax *14*
Whales 117
Wheat 44, 45, 55, *121*, *124*-126, *135*
Wheat germ oil 61
Wine *80*

Xerophthalmia 58

Yeast *64*, *65*, 128, 141, 143
Yogurt *59*, *74*, 97, 98, 132

Zinc 12, 83
Zymase 128